Dana's Last 10 Years

A play by   Michael J. Padgett

Originally written summer, 2021

Contents

Introduction to the Play

This morning for the second time in a week, I smelled Dana's mother's house. Her house always had a distinctive smell. I'm not sure if it was some sort of hand cream or a cleaning liquid.   I would always smell the same thing when I went into her parent's house. It's not a bad smell, definitely the feminine smell of an older generation. It is a smell that I link directly to Dana's mother.

Why would I start smelling it now when I come out of my girlfriend's bedroom early in the morning? I did not smell it in the house 2 weeks ago or 2 months ago. I only smell it early, as I'm heading out for a workout before dawn, when the house is still dark.

Last week was the second anniversary of Dana's mother's death. I placed new ferns around our 5 headstones, trying to make it all look less abandoned, less forlorn in an old Houston cemetery on the bank of Buffalo Bayou. Is she telling me that it is time for me to join them? She had a horrible death that still wracks my insides.

It's been a little over 2 years since the events unfolded. For me, the years may have gone by, but the sadness, guilt and horror are too much alive. A friend, Jim Meehan, who lost his wife many years ago wrote me a letter about "the void." He felt a void inside after Anne's death. His letter nailed the feeling. I still have a void. It's a void that feels as if it is centered in my chest where my heart should be. I think some part of my brain's circuitry has been blown away, leaving the ghostly feeling of a void where my heart should be, a "missing limb syndrome" of the heart. It's a real void that is filled with emptiness tinged with sadness and dark memories. It has all left me numb inside with little or no ability to enjoy things or perhaps even to feel love again.

I have been told that I have PTSD. It may be true. It is definitely true that I have a great deal of sympathy and respect for the guys who have seen horrendous things in combat. When you've seen a person that you love or care about destroyed, you can never escape the images, the events or the memories. PTSD seems like a perfectly reasonable response to horrible things.

I have been asked to convert this piece to a novel but have resisted. It came to me as a play in the months after those events. I would love to see it performed on-stage sometime. A performance might help bring Dana's story alive and help the viewer see how it applies to her life or to the lives of women in her life.

In the meantime, the purpose of this play is to show you how one woman's medical problems and interaction with the American medical establishment contributed to her death. The goal is not to cast blame, because medicine in America is evolving and in many ways is very immature. It is especially immature and imprecise when it comes to women's health.

I was once told in a physics lecture that any measurement without error bars is meaningless. Every measurement has inherent errors and without finding out the error level there is no way to determine reliability or significance. I wonder if I will ever see the results of a simple blood test with the error bars stated.

Dana once had blood samples taken at the same time sent to two different labs for thyroid hormone analysis. The results that came back differed enough to change the prescribed replacement hormone dosages. Neither lab specified "error bars" and the lack of precision meant that there was no way to assess which might be more reliable. In Dana's case, thyroid hormone replacement levels became a real driver of quality of life.

To help you get a perspective about the events of the play, a little history is in order. Dana and I met in 1982 and were married in late March of 1983. We both had finished degrees and were working as programmers for Nasa contractors in Clear Lake, Texas. She was 23 and I was 29 when we got married. At the time her parents were living in Saudi Arabia and her younger brother, Britton, was at UT-Austin. We never had children. There was a miscarriage after a number of years, but it was clear that children would never come. It is a sadness for me that we never had kids.

As the years went by, Dana's parents retired to Houston. Her brother eventually retired in Austin. He never married or had children. Britton died very unexpectedly of a probable heart event in July, 2015. None of us ever really recovered from Britton's death. For me, Britton was like a third brother. He was incredibly bright and kind. Dana's mother would sit in her chair and cry for weeks at a time. Dana's father was more stoic but grieved no less. For Dana, Britton's death left her with the loss of the one person in the world that she felt that she could really talk to, soul-to-soul. Dana's loss was huge.

The events of this play started in late February, 2021. Covid had been around for over a year, and everyone was stressed. Vaccines had been developed and we all got shots. We could almost see the end of the Covid struggle but were not at the end yet. Covid added a level of stress to everyone.

Dana and I had been married for 37 years at this point. Dana's parents were in their early 80's. Her father's health was not great, and his mobility was almost non-existent because of bad knees. Dana had an elevator installed for her father and later a generator for the elevator. Eventually, both of her parents found the elevator useful.

Dana's mother was the primary caregiver, but had a great "helper," Anthony, for part of the day. Dana's parents were coping but were not happy, at least as viewed from the outside. Financially, they were doing well but money has no meaning when health and life are under stress.

The story in the play starts with the onset of Dana's health problems, 10 years earlier. I could have started the story earlier with Dana's endometriosis or probable heart issues, but Dana was about 50 when the health issues really started to set up the dominoes. Ten years seems like the right time interval to focus on and certainly contains some definite medical events.

The play was written with as much accuracy as I could manage, but it is my telling of the story.   The other principles in the story have all been cremated. I tried to get it "on paper" while events were fresh, but any telling of a story is bound to be slanted by the author's point of view. I have a point of view that has been influenced by the events themselves. Do I wish that Dana was here to correct my misremembering? … Absolutely…. But that is part of the sadness of it all. Dana had an incredible verbal acuity.

Finally, please excuse any misspellings or bad grammar that you find. As an author, I am neither experienced nor polished. Also, if you choose to read this play, be warned that there are parts that are hard to read, and you may find them disturbing. The disturbing parts happened but I do not try to dwell on them.   Perhaps some day an editor will help focus even those events.

Michael J. Padgett,   May, 2023

(Mike is sitting at a kitchen table with 4 chairs. The narrator is either on the other side of the stage or is not visible. The narrator can only be a voice.)

Narrator: I am going to try to tell a story. It is not a rigorous report but only a story. I have never tried to tell a story before and hope that you will forgive my clumsiness. I am only doing this because it seems like a story that some people might want to hear.

Right now, Mike is sitting in the kitchen of Dana's parents' house, waiting for some estate brokers to come and begin a sales process. While he waits, perhaps I can start to explain some of what happened to Dana, also to her family.

Before I go back and start telling you about Dana's history, I need to state 2 things up-front. First, Mike honestly believes that all of the medical people who worked with Dana were acting in good faith and did the best that their skills, talents, or technologies would allow. He does not think any of them were bad people or acted with willful negligence. The second thing that I need to state up front is that Mike considers this mess to be his fault. In a few critical events, he knows that he either failed to act or did the wrong thing. So, as you listen to this story, please keep in mind that things could have turned out differently, if he had acted differently. Mike knows this. Have no doubt that he knows this.

To start this story, I need to go back 10 years to when Dana was 51 and was in full menopause.

Dana: I feel bad.

Mike: How do you mean? What kind of bad?

Dana: The anxiety is out of control. I can't stand it and the depression is dark. I hurt, my muscles are spasming all the time in my legs, my butt…in the pelvic area. The diarrhea is constant. I can't sleep. I can't stand for an hour and teach my classes. It's too much. I feel bad.

Narrator: Dana soon went on a medical leave from teaching in the Art Department at the University of Houston. The people in the department were very understanding an especially the chairman, Rex Koontz. Dana went to a sequence of doctors trying to find some relief. She started with a psychiatrist that we'll call Mary and a gynecologist that we'll call Ginnie.

Psychiatrist-Mary: We need to talk about this, about what you are feeling. Was it something your mother did when you were a teenager? The anxiety has to be coming from your life somewhere. Is it your marriage?

In the meantime, we'll start you on Xanax and keep trying different anti-depressants until we find one that works for you.

Dana: It's been 4 sessions and I still feel bad. I still hurt. My muscles are still twitching all of the time. The depression is getting worse by the day. I can't sleep. Sometimes, I only get 2 or 3 hours of sleep a night. I feel bad.

Narrator: The psychiatry was not providing any relief at all. Weeks went by and symptoms were getting worse. Dana tried the gynecological route to see if there was something that could be causing the pelvic area pain.

After the exam, the gynecologist took Dana by the shoulders, and shook her:

Gynecologist-Ginnie: I've done a full exam. There is nothing wrong with you. It is all in your head. Do you hear me? It's all in your head.

Narrator: Dana was basically thrown out by Ginnie the gynecologist. This incident stuck with her. She was getting worse and worse. It was definitely not all in her head.

Mike: They are not helping. Can you go to your doctor and just ask them to run tests? Get them to draw blood and test for everything. Just collect data.

Narrator: A week or so went by and Dana did go to her primary care doctor. She requested that they draw blood and run all of the tests that they could.

Dana: I got a call from my primary. She said that my thyroid numbers were off the chart.   I have hyper-thyroidism, Graves' disease.

Narrator: At this point, the whole episode had been going on for a couple of months. Dana had been to many psych-talk sessions and several other physicians. She was on loads of Xanax and had been through a laundry list of anti-depressants. During this whole time, none of the physicians ever ordered a blood test until Dana went in and requested it.

 Dana's TSH was .0063 and her T4-free was 3.48. Earlier when Dana was healthy, her TSH was measured at 1.89 - 2.53 which is in the normal range of .4 - 4.5 mIU/mL. Her T4-free was measured at 1.17, also in a normal range of 0.9 - 1.7 ng/dL. A TSH level of .0063 is really bad and T4-free was running at almost 3 times her healthy number.

It turns out that Dana's experience is probably typical for thyroid problems. It normally takes about 3 months to diagnose an out-of-control thyroid. The problem is that thyroid hormones control metabolism…. EVERYWHERE. The leg, butt and pelvic spasms Dana was experiencing were happening because the muscle cells were firing in overdrive, even the muscles that line the vagina. It really was everywhere. Also, thyroid problems are often first diagnosed as anxiety-depression problems….a brain out of control, in overdrive. So, Dana's 2-3 months to get a diagnosis was not that unusual.

Human beings have two primary signaling systems. Nerves carry electro-chemical impulses along definite pathways and can transmit signals in milli-seconds. It how we jerk our fingers off of a burning hot surface.

The endocrine system is a slower signaling system using chemicals called hormones. These chemicals are produced by specific cells somewhere in our bodies, put into the bloodstream and then go everywhere. They attach to the membranes of cells and tell the cells to do something. We have cells in our stomach linings that stretch when we get full. Stretching these cells, causes them to send out a chemical signal that goes to our brains to tell us to stop eating…my stomach is full now.

The thyroid hormones regulate the rate of metabolism. They are bigger molecules that can take a long time to soak into all of our tissues. For instance, it can take weeks for a change in thyroid hormone levels to fully soak into the cartilage in the joints in your fingers. It's a slow and, hopefully, steady signaling system.

The thyroid gland produces the main thyroid hormones. It is told how much to produce by the thyroid stimulating hormone, TSH. TSH is produced in the pituitary gland under the direction of the hypothalamus. When thyroid levels are high in the blood, the hypothalamus tells the pituitary to produce less TSH, which means that the thyroid should produce less Thyroid hormones, like T3 and T4.

It's all exquisitely complicated and works amazingly well so long as each piece is doing its job. It is like a bicycle. You step on the pedal, which moves the front sprocket, which moves the chain, which moves the back gears, which moves the wheel and off you go. What happens if somebody puts a stick in the spokes?

In Dana's case, something was not working right because the T4-Free level was 3 times normal at 3.48 when the TSH level was .0063. The hypothalamus was signaling to turn off hormone production, but the thyroid was going full out. Dana's thyroid hormone system was out of whack.

Grave's disease is an autoimmune disease in which an antibody is produced called a Thyroid Stimulating Immunoglobulin, TSI, an IG immunoglobulin. TSI attaches to TSH receptors on the thyroid in a way that ramps up activation, telling the thyroid to make lots more T3 and T4. TSI is not restrained by the hypothalamus-pituitary feedback loop. With lots of TSI in the blood, the hypothalamus and pituitary shut down TSH production, which means a low number while the thyroid pumps out more and more T3 and T4. Dana had an autoimmune disease that was acting like a stick in her bicycle spokes.

For Dana, then came treatment, which was by a woman who did med school at Harvard and had just finished a fellowship in women's health at Columbia. We'll call her Gamma.

Mike: I remember Gamma. She was probably mid-thirties. She was petite and always wore a pink and white dress-suit under her lab coat. She would stand in the corner of the exam room, holding her matching purse in front of her with both hands, just above the waist. She would never approach the patient, Dana in this case. Her credentials were solid, and we hoped that she would help.

Dana always deferred to her physicians and would rigorously do what they said.

Women's specialist-Gamma: Women are designed to have children and die when they are 50.

Narrator: This was a big "Wow" to say to a 50-year-old patient, but she prescribed a thyroid suppressant that had Dana feeling Ok within about 2 weeks.

Women's specialist-Gamma: The dosage of the thyroid suppressant is too high. Your numbers might go too low. We need to drop the dosage by 30%.

Narrator: One week later, Dana is back in full hyper-thyroid distress.

Women's specialist-Gamma: This is not working. We need to remove the thyroid. The recommendation here at Buxxey School of Medicine is radioactive iodine treatment. We don't want this to ever happen again, so we will use a strong dose. But, you could do surgery. It is your choice.

Mike: How do you choose? With surgery, there is the risk of cutting the nerve going to the larynx. At Buxxey, radiation is their version of a "gold standard" of treatment. Neither of us has any experience with this. How do you choose?

Later, Dana and I always referred to a "gold standard" of treatment. It's the treatment that will get you a right answer on a standardized test covering current practice in "American" medicine. I always think about poor George Washington who got the "gold standard" of treatment several times before his death. In his time, bleeding was the "gold standard," in order to drain the bad humors out of the body. At Buxxey, you get a "gold standard' of treatment.

Narrator: Dana did go with the radiation. She was later told that Gamma had prescribed a dose that was too high. For Dana, it meant that the dying thyroid was dumping 3 months of thyroid hormones into her system over the course of about 4 weeks, while it continued to make new hormones using radioactive iodine. Hyper-thyroidism became cataclysmic thyroidism. Dana's symptoms went off the charts again during a Houston August.

Mike: That August was the first escape to Colorado. I drew a circle on the map to find the closest cool weather to Houston. Denver is slightly over a 2-hour flight. With another 90 minutes in the car, you can be up into cool air. I booked a trip to Breckenridge and found a place called Beaver Run, a condo complex with a restaurant.

It wasn't clear that Dana could make the trip. She could barely walk to the plane. She was exhausted and still out of her mind with the anxiety and depression, but we made it.

The first trip to Beaver Run was just desperation. We would get up in the morning and have breakfast in the restaurant. Dana could walk during the day and then we would have dinner out some place. The ski runs at Breckenridge are all weed covered swaths through the forest in the summer. Just across a ski run from Beaver Run is the Burro Trail. It starts at a footbridge over a stream and then goes up by the stream for half a mile or so. The stream gurgles all the way up and the walk through the forest can be amazingly restful. It was a good first walk in Breckenridge and I think helped Dana to start recovering from the thyroid storm.

(Show Dana and Mike hiking.)

Narrator: Over the next 10 years, they would take many trips to Colorado. They always went back to Breckenridge in Summitt County. Breckenridge is at about 9300 feet with about 33% less oxygen than down in Houston. The first few days there, breathing would always be a little difficult, but it would be much cooler than Houston or even Denver. Dana could not take the heat anymore. Sometimes, she would dump sweat instantly and passed out on a couple of occasions.

The hiking with its deep breathing worked for Dana. All she had to worry about was her shoes, backpack, water, and trail mix. Walking in the deep woods always calmed her. Over the years, they would walk and later bicycle literally hundreds of miles in the Summitt County area. Anxiety, depression, and health are why they traveled to the high country, but there is more to this.

(Show Dana and Mike sitting on a rock drinking from water bottles.)

Mike: We stayed a few days until I needed to call a doctor for a temperature and Dana had a strange breathing event early in the morning. She made a raspy-gasping breathing sound and would not wake up. I shook her and called to her. Eventually, she started breathing normally and kind of came around. I don't remember if she threw up, but the effects lasted awhile.

The doctor made a "house call" with a bottle of oxygen in his bag. We told him what was going on and what happened with Dana. He said we were both just suffering from the altitude. It did cut the trip short but was better than baking in Houston.

Narrator: That first trip to Breckenridge helped Dana get through the catastrophe of the thyroid storm after irradiation, but it did not solve the thyroid problem. With no thyroid hormones, a person soon has their metabolism slow to the point of death. The hormones must be replaced.
At Buxxey Medical School, the replacement philosophy was one of strict replacement by T4 and nothing else. The theory is that you replace the T4 with a synthetic like Levoxyl, and the body

converts it to T3 and then everything works fine. T3 is the metabolite that is a used within cells to determine the rate of metabolism. You use blood tests to monitor TSH, T3 and T4 levels in the blood to determine how much of the replacement hormones to give somebody. A normally functioning thyroid is producing T3 and T4 at a rate of 20% T3 and 80% T4.

In Dana's case, they kept giving her more and more T4 supplement but the T3 level barely budged. In fact, they gave her so much T4 that many of the old hyper-thyroid symptoms returned.

Mike: I started keeping a log of Dana's symptoms on a day-by-day basis, assigned a numerical value to the severities and plotted versus the prescribed T4 dosages. It became clear at what dosage the symptoms would take off. When you plotted T4 dose versus measured T4-Free and TSH 3 in the blood, it also became clear that you would kill Dana before you would hit a T4 Free or T3 target. A single supplement did not work for her. Her T4-to-T3 conversion system did not work correctly after the radiation. I tried to show the graphs to some of her endocrinologists, but these guys clearly were not into data analysis. I don't think t they had any idea what a regression is or why anyone would do one. The idea of using a multi-linear fit to determine a dosage level was nothing that they wanted any part of.

It turns out that the kind of plots that I was doing have a history in medical literature. You can find published plots dating back to 1992 showing the relationship between TSH and T4-Free. Still for Dana, none of this made any difference.

Narrator: Dana tried a sequence of endocrinologists, at least one of them was a renowned, published author. All of them used a single T4 supplement system. They would up the dosage and then drive Dana out of her mind, one more time…...which meant more Xanax and anti-depressants from Mary, the psychiatrist.

Mike: Eventually, someone recommended a private practice doctor named Arem. He did not take insurance, but some people seemed to have luck with him. I think he may have been North African originally and was definitely not tied to the Buxxey School of Medicine approach or their "Gold Standard" of treatment.

I went with Dana on one of her first visits. The waiting area was filled with about a dozen women waiting and one man. That seemed about right since thyroid problems are 12 times more common in women than in men.

Arem listened to Dana. He would ask how she felt. I don't think he ever told her how she should feel or that what she was feeling was in her head. He actually listened to the patient before deciding what the patient's problems were. He never once took her by the shoulders and told her that there was nothing wrong with her, but he did say that the radiation dose given her by the faculty member of Buxxey was too high.

Arem always drew blood and always used the same lab for thyroid hormone analysis. This gave him consistency from one visit to the next. Using the lab numbers and what he heard from Dana, he would adjust dosages…...in exceedingly small increments.

I have to add that he also used more than just a T4 supplement. He prescribed Armour Thyroid which the Buxxey School of Medicine clan would not touch, not part of the "gold standard." Armour Thyroid is ground-up, desiccated animal thyroid gland. This means that it contains not just T4, but also T3, T1, T2, T6, T7 and all the other T's that a functioning thyroid makes. A rough set of numbers that I found indicated that 0.5 grain (30 mGm) of Armour would have about 12.5 μGm of T3 + 50 μGm of T4, a similar ratio to a functioning thyroid gland, 4-to-1.

Mixing the standard T4 supplement with small amounts of Armour Thyroid finally allowed Dana's numbers to approach the target of both T4-Free and TSH in "normal ranges." As soon as her numbers got better for both, all of the other symptoms, including the anxiety and depression, got better. This was about two years from when all of this began.

Narrator: With Dana's thyroid numbers getting slowly in-line, she began to live more normally by taking thyroid supplements twice a day. Dana was rigorous about timing and taking the supplements on an empty stomach.

(Show plot on a screen if it helps the story. See Supplemental Material.)

During all this time, she was still going to Mary the psychiatrist for "talk therapy." Dana was taking heavy doses of Xanax and then Prozac for the corresponding depression. For Dana, as a dose of Xanax would wear off, the depression would build in.

Mike: During the first years 4 years of the thyroid, anxiety, depression phase, I was trying to hold down a job. At that time, the job involved travel to LA. I cannot count the number of times that I talked to Dana over the phone from LAX before boarding with the anxiety and depression absolutely raging. She would talk about being in a dark place many times. I would get home late at night and wonder if Dana would still be alive. I'd go upstairs and check…. Still breathing….OK….home.

Narrator: Dana kept going to Mary because she was absolutely addicted to Xanax and maybe Prozac. Dana had to keep going and paying because Mary was her supplier. She wrote the prescriptions. She was her pusher.

Mike: Being on prescription drugs really bothered Dana and she said so, more than once. She had always been a healthy independent woman. The drugs and addiction brought into question every concept that she had of herself. She hated being an addict, but slowly started to wean herself off the Xanax. It took several years to get off the Xanax. She was probably on Xanax for at least 6-7 years. She never actually weaned herself off the Prozac. The Prozac instantly went away one afternoon after the fifth cardiac incident.

Narrator: Before getting into the cardiology, we need to go back and look at the younger Dana so that you can get a feel for what kind of woman she was. Dana did a degree in Computer Engineering at Vanderbilt and then took a job writing code for Computer Science Corporation in Clear Lake, at the Johnson Space Center. She started by writing orbital propagators for the Space Shuttle Flight Design System. A propagator took a state vector, like location and orientation of the shuttle, and moved it around an orbit one time step at a time, like from one hundredth of a second to the next hundredth of a second.

Dana met Mike in a computer room in Building 30, the old Mission Control Building. He was also writing code for the Flight Design System for another NASA contractor. Their first date was iced tea at the old NASA cafeteria in the middle of the afternoon. Dana thought this was really racy.

(Show Mike and Dana off the side drinking iced tea.)

One incident from that time is telling. One of Dana's supervisors would come up behind her and rub her shoulders. She asked him to stop. He didn't. So, she turned to him:

Dana: Do that again and I'll break your arm.

Narrator: He left her alone.

Mike: Dana had the largest, most beautiful eyes that I have ever seen. She was stunningly beautiful. She was smart and was willing to sail with me on a 470 on Galveston Bay or go snorkeling in Cozumel. She had almost no furniture in her apartment, but her apartment was home for her younger brother when he came for a visit from UT. We would sit on the floor to watch TV or have dinner. It didn't seem bad to me or to her brother, Britton.

When I met Dana, Britton was studying Mechanical Engineering at UT Austin. During his freshman year, their parents moved to Saudi Arabia with Aramco. Britton's home-base left the country after his parents sold the things he grew up with. Dana's father was the manager at Ras Tanura, which at that time was the largest refinery in the world. He was officially a Texaco employee temporarily working for Aramco. Dana liked having her parents 9 time zones away, but I think, Britton felt a little abandoned. Dana was his anchor. He was someone that she could talk to more comfortably than anyone else. Like Dana, Britton was a truly kind soul.

Narrator: Dana and Mike were married when she was 23 and he was 29. By then, Mike had changed to a research geophysics job with a small oil company called Getty which was later acquired by Texaco. When they were first married, Dana was still working for CSC and commuting to Clear Lake. She hated commuting.

Dana: "It's stupid to spend your life working for somebody else." In a year or so after we got married, I went back to grad school and got an MFA in painting from the University of Houston. Later, I taught, mostly art history and contemporary topics for many years. It was all adjunct teaching at UofH or one of the community colleges. Although, for a while I was teaching enough at UofH to be called "full time" with benefits. Overall, art and teaching were a much better fit for me than the computer science.

Gael Stack: My name is Gael Stack. I'm a Houston artist and was one of Dana's professors on the studio side at UofH. Many years ago, I argued to hire Dana.   I told the group, "She knows things." The art historians were being total assholes about the fact that she had an MFA and not a PhD. On the studio side, the MFA is the terminal degree. So, we hired her to teach "Contemporary Painting" as a "Studio Course." The art historians thought that nothing done in the last 50 years was art. "Contemporary Art" wasn't really art. They could just call it "Current Events," or whatever, as far as I was concerned.

We required all the studio students to take Dana's course. She put together a course that no one could match. When she finally quit, the studio coordinator wanted her notes and slides. She reluctantly gave them away, but still, no one could teach "Contemporary Painting" the way she did. She had too much depth. When she quit, I think we were the losers.

Dana and Mike lived two doors down from me, so I could keep up with Dana, even when her problems started. We would walk and talk and meet for coffee. Mike would bake and we traded lots of food over 3 decades.

Mike: Dana and I never had kids. Let's just say that after thousands of dollars in treatments, the biology did not work out. There was a miscarriage along the way, but no more than that. I am sorry that kids never happened, and I still wonder if Dana was sorry also. Britton never married and so there were never any grandkids for Dana's parents. I throw this in to give a bit more context before picking up the story again.

Dana: During the years before "The Troubles," we lived a quiet life. We renovated an old house and did most of the work ourselves. Mike had worked in construction to help pay for undergrad. He knew how to make a concrete form, put up a stud wall, how to wire, how to fix plumbing, really most things, but was no good at caulking or painting. He could not paint a toothpick without getting paint all over himself and the floor. Still, the house turned out well although there are still projects to do.

We would travel every year. Normally, we'd go to New York in
the Fall, go to galleries, to museums and try new restaurants. Mike
and I both liked walking in Central Park. We did a couple of
longer trips. Most all of the trips were active, and we would walk
a huge amount.

With Britton, we did a lot of bike riding. Later, he even came up
to Breckenridge and we rode the bike paths and even pedaled up to
Vail Pass.

I had always been a lap swimmer. Mike and I did lots of things
around water. In my early 40's, I started surfing. Mike had started
when he was a kid in San Diego. Then, one day we were at a surf
shop in Houston and there was a red pin-tail Gary Linden for sale.
We bought it and I started learning from Mike. The first few
lessons were rough because the waves at Surfside were too small.
At one point, Mike said, "Just throw yourself on the board," which
became a running joke. Eventually, I got better, and we started
taking the boards to San Diego in the summer. Gary Linden made
a new board for me, and it was my main board from then on.
People don't think there is any surf in Texas but there is a place
where the sand shelf is building, and the waves can be great on a
good day. One day, Mike and I both took off on the same wave
and a dolphin swam in the wave between us. The water, the beach,
coral, fish, surfing, swimming…. would always help me.

I got into triathlons for a while and did the Dove all women's
triathlon in Austin for several years. Mike would take a board up
to the lake and help with the water safety. Britton would help with
bicycles around the course. My parents would drive up for the
race. The Dove Triathlons became outings for the whole family.
Really, until "The Troubles," I was healthy. We were active.

Narrator: There is at least one study in the literature that says that
it takes about 5 years for someone to recover fully from thyroid
oblation using radioactive iodine. For Dana, it was 4-5 years

before the thyroid had settled down and she was able to get decrease the Xanax to a low dose, but not the Prozac. By the Spring of the fifth year, there had been many trips to Colorado and even discussions about buying a second home. In late March, a trip was planned to go back to Colorado to inspect a property that Mike and Dana had made an offer on. Dana was feeling anxious around the decision and was still on a low dose of Xanax and on Prozac. Then there was another early morning breathing incident, the third one.

Mike: That morning in early March could have turned out differently. Like the time in Breckenridge, I woke up with Dana doing a raspy gasping, gagging kind of sound, trying to catch a breath. I said, "Dana, wake up." She was unresponsive and her eyes were fixed, staring like a dead dog. I thought it was a breathing problem. I rolled her onto her left side and used the fingers of my left hand to clear her throat. She had swallowed her tongue. Then, with my right hand, I pushed up from her stomach up into her diaphragm, trying to move air. I kept repeating, "Dana, wake up." I was afraid she would not wake up, but eventually she took a breath. We got her sitting up and then she threw up.

After she stabilized some, I called the Psychiatrist-Mary. I explained about the raspy-gagging sound, the trying to breath and the dead dog stare. She just said maybe I should call an ER. She was no help or even acknowledge that this could be serious…basically, nothing.

So, I called an ER and talked to an ER doc. I told him the same story and he said maybe next time I should immediately take her to an ER, but for now, nothing to do.

Dana slowly gained strength as the day went on, but she was really weak and kind of rattled. The doctors in Houston were of no use.

Narrator: Dana and Mike did make the trip to Colorado to look at a property up in French Gulch. It became clear to Mike that Dana did not want to buy it. This was some sort of fantasy of his. They declined on the property and went back to Houston where things were stable until July.

(Two Houston Police officers in uniform at a front gate. 9:00 pm)

Houston Police Officer 1 of 2: Are you Dana Padgett? You are listed as the contact person for Britton Birmingham in Austin. I have the Travis County Medical Examiner on the line.

Narrator: Dana took the call. Britton was found dead in his bed earlier that morning by Ray, his neighbor across the street. There was no foul play, probably his heart. The medical examiner would not know anything more until after the autopsy. She and Mike were stunned. Mike would later say that the 2 HPD officers did an amazingly good and kind job in handling this. It was July 17, 4 and a half years after Dana's troubles began.

Mike: Dana decided to call her mother and tell her. Dana's mother did not sleep that night and never really recovered from the death of her only son. We went to their house the next morning. The shock and sadness were infinite. Later, we went with them to the funeral home, to the cemetery to buy a plot for the family, to place his ashes, order a headstone and do all of the rest.

After a while, we went to Austin and met with Britton's neighbors. Ray and Jan across the street hosted a remembrance for all the neighbors. Britton lived in Hyde Park, just north of UT. It was a small community of people, of neighbors who cared for him and he for them. That Britton lived around people who cared for him gave comfort to Dana, and I hope to her parents. He had left everything to Dana, and she handled all the paperwork around his affairs, never easy. The loss of Britton was huge for Dana, just huge.

He was a great friend, incredibly smart and a kind soul. He made a bicycle for me and gave Dana a road bike. I can not guess the number of miles that we three biked together. He helped us work on our house in Houston and we would help work on his in Austin. For Dana, whenever she needed a kind ear, she'd call Britton. Thanksgiving and Christmas without Britton, how could that be?

Narrator: To get away from Houston for a while and the heat of late August, Mike and Dana went back to Breckenridge just before Labor Day. They hiked a couple of days and looked at a couple of houses with a realtor. On the Sunday before Labor Day, they were supposed to look at another house.

Mike: Like the last time in Houston, in March, I woke up with Dana doing a raspy, gasping, gagging kind of trying to catch a breath sound. I said, "Dana, wake up." She was unresponsive and her eyes were fixed, staring like a dead dog again. I still thought it was a breathing problem. I rolled her onto her left side and used the fingers of my left hand to clear her throat. She had swallowed her tongue, like in Houston. Then, with my right hand, I pushed up from her stomach, up into her diaphragm, trying to move air, while keeping up the "Dana, wake up." I was afraid she would not wake up and that I'd have to tell her mother that her other child had died. Eventually she took a breath. We got her sitting up and then she threw up.

Dana: Something is wrong. I need to get to a doctor.

Mike: I called the front desk at Beaver Run and the guy on duty called an ambulance. The Summitt County ambulance guys showed up in a few minutes, hooked up Dana for heart monitoring and took her to the ER in Frisco, Colorado. These guys were extremely efficient.

I got to the ER in Frisco. She was in an exam room wired up for a cardiac check-up. She looked stunned and pale. The young ER doc, Stephen Altmin, was a guy from Australia who normally worked rescue in the Himalayas. He was working Frisco in the "off-season," down at 9000 ft.

I caught up with Dr. Altmin in he hallway.

ER-S. Altmin: Do you know how to read an EKG?

Mike: Not really.

Er-S. Altmin: OK, I found something odd in her strip. I think it could be something with her heart.

Mike: Her younger brother just died suddenly, 6 weeks ago. Nothing definitive, but the speculation is that it was his heart.

Er-S. Altmin: OK, she needs to go to Denver to see a real cardiologist. We don't have what she needs here.

Mike: When and where?

Er-S. Altmin: As soon as I can arrange it. She will go to the Adventist Hospital in Littleton. She'll be transported by ambulance.

Mike: Can I go with her?

Er-S. Altmin: No, you can catch up to her there.

Mike: I went in and told Dana what was going on and that I'd see her at the hospital in Littleton. Next, I checked us out of Beaver Run, told the receptionist for the realtor that we would not be able to make our appointment later and drove to the hospital in Littleton.

Narrator: Stephen Altmin in Frisco had detected a long QT interval, which is why he knew something unusual was going on. He was the first doctor to ever check an EKG after one Dana's events. Mike and Dana were convinced that Altmin had kept her alive.

They transported Dana by ambulance from Frisco to Littleton, keeping her sitting up the whole time. She left Frisco at about 11:20 in the morning. They didn't give her anything to eat or drink. In Littleton, the on-call cardiologist for the pre-Labor Day weekend was an old cardiologist named Harvey Schuchman. He was a guy who had seen many things. They got her in a room and wired her up. She was having intermittent VTACH from about 1:00 pm: Her QT interval was measured at .537 seconds, just about the time Mike arrived.

Mike: I arrived at Dana's room in Littleton about 2:55 pm and said hello to the cardiologist. I stood at the end of the bed. They lowered Dana back to a prone position. She immediately went into full VFib/VTACH. The cardiologist was standing next to the bed. He called a code-zero and the room filled up with people. There must have been 2 dozen people in the room. Schuchman started doing chest compressions until the cart arrived. I started to think that if they did not get her back soon, I would need to step in and do my tongue-and-breathing procedure.

Schuchman: Is it charged? Shock her … damn it … shock her.

Narrator: They gave her 120 joules plus magnesium. Schuchman wrote it up as "ventricular tachycardia as well as torsades de pointes."

(Project strips on the wall. They are copied at the end of this document, in the Appendices).

Narrator: It took them a solid 3 minutes to bring Dana back. You can see the strips there. A nurse later said, "Can we use your strips? It is textbook. We've never seen anybody come back from that." Out in the hallway, the cardiologist was calming down. He was rattled and was talking to his electrician-cardiologist colleague, Choe. Mike joined them.

Mike: I told him: "That is what happened in Breckenridge this morning." He wanted to know how I got her out of it and rapidly explained my procedure.

Schuchman: What are you?

Mike: Mostly a geophysicist but I studied physics.

Schuchman: Do you see these strips? This is not consistent with life.

(Show the EKG traces in the middle of the series.)

Cardiologist-Choe: What is she taking, what medicines?

Mike: She is on thyroid supplements for Graves' disease, Xanax for anxiety and Prozac.

Cardiologist-Choe: Prozac? That stops today.

Narrator: They wheeled Dana off to the Cath-lab and put in a temporary pacemaker. This was Dana's fifth cardiac event. Later in the room, the Cardiologist-Choe came by.

Cardiologist-Choe: You have Long-QT syndrome. Basically, the QT interval is the time at the end of a heartbeat when the ventricular part of your heart is giving up potassium as electrical charge. It has to depolarize before starting another beat. If it takes too long and the next beat starts before the last beat is finished uncharging, then ventricular fibrillation happens. The heart muscles are firing chaotically. The heart stops pumping or moving blood. So, there is no circulation to anything, including the brain.

Narrator: A Long QT V-fib/VTACH event like Dana's has a mortality rate of 90-95%. Long QT Syndrome is normally detected in younger people because they either have an event and die or someone is sharp when reviewing an EKG. In Dana's case, it was a sharp ER doc in Frisco who noticed a problem. It is interesting that he was the first one to catch anything. In Dana's first cardiac event when she was in her 30's, she went to the ER and the guy said that it was probably either the flu or her time of the month.

Mike: None of the doctors ever commented on the gasping-raspy trying to catch a breath thing. It's called, "Agonal Breathing." It is a deep brain stem response when blood flow has ceased, and the rest of the brain is off-line. It's a very primitive brain-stem level reflex. Did any of these doctors get taught what Agonal Breathing sounds like? …. When coupled with a dead-dog eye stare?

Narrator: Long QT is genetic and there are known genetic markers. Dana was tested and her DNA test came back positive for Long QT. Britton was never tested.

There are drugs that can induce an event. In each of the events that Dana experienced, she was on one of those drugs, even the first one when she was in her 30's. Prozac is on the list, but so is Benadryl and some antibiotics. There is a website call CredibleMeds that Dana checked carefully after getting out of the hospital. How many young people die in their beds every year because genetically they are pre-disposed to Long QT and then get prescribed something? Their friends and parents will never know why they just died.

Cardiologist-Choe: You cannot leave this hospital without an implanted pacemaker/defibrillator. Tomorrow is Labor Day. We cannot get one put in until Tuesday. In the meantime, try to stay still.

Mike: At this point, Dana was in a Cardiac ICU bed. She had a temporary pacemaker threaded up her femoral artery. She could not move very much but did once and the wire shifted. It caused her heart rhythm to go squirrely. One of the nurses brought in a portable defibrillator and put it on the tray table next to her bed. It was spooky to understand what was going on.

Later that day, I called Dana's parents to tell them some of what I knew. Dana's mother wanted to know if she needed to come to Denver immediately. I told her that I thought Dana was stable, meaning that she did not need to come to Denver and say, "Goodbye."

Narrator: They implanted an ICD on Tuesday and kept Dana a little longer for observation.

Cardiologist-Choe: With your condition and the ICD, you cannot get on a ladder, you can not drive, and you can not swim. If you have another event, you will lose consciousness before the defibrillator shocks you back. These activities are too dangerous for you now.

Dana: Can I hike at altitude or bicycle or something?

Cardiologist-Choe: They should be mostly OK. The unit is designed to increase your heart rate when you exercise.

Mike: Mostly, we thought that the guys at South Denver Cardiology did a good job. The care at the Adventist Hospital in Littleton seemed much more competent than we had seen in Houston. Dana felt that she was just lucky that the ER doc in

Frisco was the one to see her. She believed that if some other physician had just sent her back to Beaver Run "to relax," then she might have just died that afternoon.

Narrator: Mike was able to arrange a flight back to Houston and later that week, they made it home. Dana was still sore from the device installation and especially from the chest compressions that first day in Littleton. Chest compressions hurt.

Back in Houston, a friend, Kathy Hall, whose husband had been a surgeon, was able to get a recommendation for a local cardiologist to take on her case. His name was Miguel Valderrabano of the DeBakey group. He did med school in Spain and Dana always found him to be focused and interested. A few years later, he had to replace an atrial lead and Dana thought that he did an exceptionally good job at placing the ICU back and stitching up the incision.

After they returned, Dana and Mike went to Dana's parents' house to show them that she was still around. They were relieved and said, "Thank you" to Mike.

Dana had 2 new health things. First, Dana now had to take some cardiac meds in addition to her thyroid supplements. It bothered her that she was now someone who had a closet full of bottles, but she kept up with it. The other thing that changed was that now there was a transmitter in the bedroom that would communicate with her ICD every night and transmit to the mother ship every morning about 2:00 am. The idea was that if there were an event, Valderrabano would get an alert. He also had a history printed out every time that she went to see him after that.

Dana also checked in with a new internist that thought a lot of.

Internist-Matus: You were dead. What did you see?

Dana: What do you mean?

Internist-Matus: Did you see angels or your grandparents or what?

Dana: I didn't see anything. When I came back, I was just back, but before, nothing.

Internist-Matus: Nothing?

Dana: Nothing.

Mike: Dana had been through 5 of these cardiac events. She believed that she had experienced death and returned. Dana believed absolutely that with death there was just nothingness …. just nothing.

(Turn off the house lights.)

Dana would have called herself an agnostic with respect to God but fully believed that with death there was just nothing. By this point, she had absolutely no fear of death. If you are a theologian, you can argue that she never really died. You can argue that her "soul" never left her body. Maybe that's true, but Dana believed that she had experienced death and was sure that when she "died" other people might go on, but for her nothing. There was no heaven or hell, just nothingness.

(Turn house lights back on.)

(Intermission)

Narrator: After Dana settled in with the ICD and was able to get wet, she immediately went back to lap swimming and yoga. The lap swimming was her way to calm her mind and maintain her sanity. She completely ignored the instructions of the

Cardiologist-Choe in Denver. For her, giving up lap swimming would mean that she would lose her sanity immediately.

Mike: In the years after the ICD implantation, I kind of "retired' after a job with Signal Hill Petroleum in Long Beach went away. The guys at Signal Hill had been amazingly understanding and kind to me.   The management there, Brady Barto, Craig Barto and Dave Slater, were way more generous with me than would have been possible in a big company. The kindness of management and colleagues has meant the world and that applies not just to Signal Hill but to my entire working career. I worked with so many smart, professional, and truly kind people that I really do feel privileged. Besides, doing oil and gas work allowed me to study the earth and learn things that I never would have learned if I had stayed in academic physics.

Narrator: Dana and Mike continued to travel, hike and swim but only in the Western Hemisphere. There were a couple of trips to St. Croix, to Belize, to the Vancouver area and to lots of national parks. The trips were the times when Dana could escape from background medical issues and a low-level anxiety that never went away. She always had a glass of wine with dinner after she finally managed to get off of the Xanax. This seemed to help her get through the night. Mike was drinking less and less and then not at all. He said the alcohol made his head hurt.

Dana: During the years after getting the ICD, the lap swimming was my only way to keep the anxiety in check. There was always a low level of anxiety just below the surface and the thyroid meds probably never really worked entirely. I had years where I hurt all of the time, like in the joints in my fingers. Joint pain is a low thyroid symptom.   Still, it was better than "The Troubles."

I told Mike that I did not fear death. I had done that and knew what to expect. The thing I feared more than anything else was ever going through "The Troubles" again. The anxiety, the depression, the pain, and the addiction are more than I could bear again. I would kill myself first.

Mike: I knew she was serious. I knew that she was completely certain about knowing what to expect after death. She feared the anxiety and depression. She hated being a Xanax-antidepressant addict. I knew she was serious, but with the thyroid largely under control, I didn't think it would ever become an issue.

Narrator: During this time, Dana's parents were getting older, more dependent, and frail, but still trying to live independently in their own house. Dana's mother fell and broke her arm while Dana and Mike were in Austin. They came back to Houston. Dana nursed and bathed her mother until she recovered.

Dana's father's health was going down steadily. Several years earlier, as his knees were getting bad, he decided that it was too risky to have knee replacements. By this time, his knees were so bad that he could barely stand. He could only use a walker by sitting on the seat and scooching around backward. The mobility problems ultimately shrank his world to the second floor of their house.

His heart had several blockages that were deemed inoperable. Invasive cardiac surgery on a man in his mid-80's is not always prudent.

Dana's father had a corkscrew esophagus. This meant that solid food ceased making it into his stomach. He would try to swallow it, and in a few minutes, it would come back up. After a couple of treatments to try to un-kink his esophagus, it was decided that this was part of his fate. The soft/fluid diet that he ate meant that he lost about 50 pounds over a 2-year period.

Dana's father was also diagnosed with pre-cancerous stomach polyps. They were deemed inoperable because of his cardiac condition. The assumption was that he would succumb to something else before the stomach would be an issue.

Dana's father also had a familial tremor in his hands that made eating with a fork almost impossible. It also meant that using a keyboard and mouse with his computer was a constant struggle. With the tremor, Dana's father really could button click faster than his computer could respond, process, or try to execute. Mike and Dana would get weekly or monthly phone calls to come out and de-scramble his computer. Sometimes, Dana's father would try to de-scramble his compute himself….not good. Mike would normally be able to do a quick reboot into safe mode, do a clean shut-down and then a fresh restart.

Finally, Dana's father's mind was slowing down, and he knew it. He wore diapers for incontinence that really bothered Dana's mother. Overall, the last few years were a struggle for a man, and his wife, who had been so capable and powerful in their prime.

Texaco-colleague: I knew Dana's father, Guy, from working at Texaco. Fast forward back to 1997 when my wife Pat and I both retired from our respective Elementary School Teacher, and Process (Refinery and Petrochemical Plant) Design Engineer, jobs. During that interval, I put in a lot of miles and time away from my family in Houston. Pat couldn't very well leave their young children, or later ask her School Principal for time off to travel with her husband, when he was working in interesting places. I felt badly, but I needed the job and the modest pay.

After 1997, I provided part-time Gasification and Flare System Consulting Services to Texaco and their Licensee Clients. Each Consulting Assignment entailed technical preparation in Houston, followed by travel to Offices and Refineries in the US, Europe, and Asia … for 1-2 weeks in each location. Pat now traveled with me, and we did a lot of local sightseeing before and after each onsite job. We were spending the consulting income on vacations!

One such assignment was at Texaco's Pembroke Refinery in Wales, UK, while Guy was the Plant Manager. Before checking into the King's Inn in Pembroke, Pat and I traveled around Wales for a week. In well-worn jeans and hiking boots, we walked mountain trails in Snowdonia, toured a Slate Mine, and hiked coastal trails from Aberystwyth to Milford Haven. I brought Nomex Safety Clothing to wear in the Refinery, and not much else. After the Consulting, we planned to walk additional coastal trails around Swansea, Port Talbot, and Cardiff.

While I was at the Refinery, Guy asked me to come to his office. We didn't have much time to chat … we both had people waiting. So Guy and Dot invited Pat and I to visit over dinner at the Bishop's Palace a few nights later. He said they would pick us up in their blue? Texaco supplied BMW. And he clued me in that Tie & Jacket, and a Dress, were required for admission to the Bishop's Palace. How could I say "No"?

I never told Guy this part of the story. After work, Pat & I hurriedly searched around Pembroke for suitable clothes. There weren't any good stores … mostly Used or Recycled shops. Pat bought new Panty Hose at a Druggist. Pat picked up a skirt, and I got slacks/shirt/tie/sport jacket, at 2-3 Used Clothing shops. Pat took the bus to Milford Haven to buy shoes … which she never wore again. But we were dressed when Guy and Dot picked us up and were admitted to the upscale Restaurant.

During the dinner conversation, Guy provided a commentary on Pembrokeshire … mostly complementary. However, he told about the "down-side" of Russian Tankers frequently docking in Milford Haven to discharge Crude Oil for the two local Refineries. The Russian Sailors swarmed the City streets, buying up huge plastic sacks of used clothing to take back home for resale. Guy said that for Russian families to actually be happy to buy and wear such "ragged clothing", was "absolutely appalling!" Pat and I looked at each other, and we almost "gagged" to keep from laughing! Little did Guy and Dot know they were dining elbow-to-elbow with such "ragged clothing" in the elegant Bishop's Palace. I never told Guy how we got dressed for their kind dinner invitation.

Dana: As my Mom and Dad got into their 80's, I struggled with how to help them. Nothing was easy. They resisted grab bars. Then my father broke the toilet in the master bathroom leaning on it. It leaked onto the living room ceiling downstairs. Then they let me put a grab bar in the bathroom, then the steps from the garage, in a second bathroom, then the shower. It was a fight to get them to accept even a shower sprayer on a hose. Then they both used it.

When my father could not get up or down stairs, I convinced them to put in an elevator. Their house had been originally designed with that in mind. It was a struggle, then both of them used it.

Because the power in their neighborhood was flaky, we got them to install a generator. Everything was a struggle.

My mother would make trays of food to take up to my father. He was constantly rejecting food that she made, saying it didn't taste good. My mother was an excellent cook. She was making soups or stews that they had eaten for years, but now they didn't taste the same. It really bothered her.

A couple of years ago, as my father got more and more wobbly, they hired a helper, Anthony, to come in 6 hours a day, 5 days a week. He had helped a couple across the street when the husband was declining.

Anthony would help my father bathe and dress in the morning, bring him breakfast and eventually lunch as well. My father did not move without Anthony by his side. Anthony managed his meds, diapers, helped with sheets that had to be washed every day. He took a huge load off of my mother.

Mike: Even with Anthony, it was clear that the whole situation was fragile. Dana's mother still wrote checks for the bills and resisted the idea of doing any "AutoPay" on accounts. Dana's mother did the shopping, banking, and errands. She still made Dana's father's supper and brought it upstairs on a tray, then picked up the tray and cleaned up. When Dana's father rejected something, it really did bother her. We tried to convince her that it was his tasting circuits and nothing she could fix, but it bothered her anyway. She tried and all of the strain exhausted her.

Narrator: During these years, Dana took on a more active role in helping to manage her parents' affairs. She was given "Power of Attorney" on their accounts and for medical decisions. Their wills were updated after Britton's death. Mike was added as secondary PoA or executor always in line after Dana. This was a new thing.

Mike: Dana and Britton always interfaced with their parents, and I always stayed out of the way. Dana's parents were kind and generous to me, but I was definitely the son-in-law and not a blood relative. That was OK with me. I could stay in the background and let Dana take the lead in all matters of importance.

Dana and I both tried to be deferential to their wishes and to accommodate them, even as their abilities declined. Dana's parents gave her static because they thought she was trying too hard. She was trying to fulfill a role that they both wanted and did not want. It's like they knew that they needed help and wanted their daughter to do things, but still did not want Dana's help. It is hard to explain how we all think differently as we get older.

Part of this developed after Britton died. Dana's mother told me that it wasn't supposed to turn out this way.

Dana's mother: Guy was supposed to die first…not Britton. It's like Guy doesn't seem to feel the loss. He doesn't express any sadness.

Mike: I am sure that after Britton died, Dana's mother just wanted to die. She stopped walking around the area. She ate lots of hamburgers and junk food. She turned down offers from Dana to go to lunch or to let us bring something over. Also, she started treating Dana's father with a harshness that really put him down, almost anytime he said anything. She hated his coughing, his mental decline, his throwing food up and the incontinence. She resented his living when Britton was gone. She hated her life.

Narrator: About this this time, the Covid-19 pandemic hit. Mike and Dana went into lockdown along with everybody else. Dana sewed masks for Mike, for herself and for her parents. Since Mike was over 65, Dana did the shopping. Mike would cook anything she brought home. They ate well, but life was stressfully abnormal. The YMCA pools shut down. Dana could not swim or go to yoga for months. Eventually, the Y started a system of reserving a swimming lane 72 hours in advance. Both Dana and Mike became regulars again.

Mike: A piece of Dana's health that I'll talk about now was her background pain. The thyroid supplements worked fairly well, but she was in almost constant pain in her joints and back. Joint pain can be a symptom of low thyroid levels. Her hand and finger pain were bad enough that she could not use a hammer. The jarring from hammering a nail hurt too much. All of the renovation that we had done years before would have impossible now.

Dana: I hurt all of the time and it makes it hard to sleep. The joints in my hands hurt. My back and shoulders hurt. I just hurt all of the time.

Mike: The background pain had been there on-and-off for years. If it was thyroid related, no one, even Arem, was able to do anything about it.

One thing started happening before the pandemic hit. Dana started using more and more Post It notes over time. She would write reminders and stick them on door jambs around the house. After forgetting about a wine bottle cooling in the freezer that froze, exploded in the freezer and I cleaned up, there were more Post It notes.

Eventually, the Post-It notes phenomena changed into more forgetfulness and confusion when driving. Dana would miss turns or not really know the way to a place that she used to go to all of the time. She was still good with her phone, but computer tasks started to seem more of a problem. There was a downward trend, and I was convinced that we would be moving to some sort of assisted living within 5 years.

I thought that Dana's mental decline was likely due to the cumulative time that she was without oxygen during the cardiac events. That is possible. Dana's cousin, Paige, and her husband, both physical therapists, pointed out that it could have been from small strokes. It could also have been from the cumulative effects of anxiety and stress over ten years. I'll never know what caused it, but it was happening, and Dana knew it.

Dana: It's starting to be hard to be around people, socially. I ca not find words. I can't be part of a conversation.

Narrator: Texas had a big, late February freeze that messed up Houston. It knocked out the pumps in the outdoor YMCA swimming pool. There were several days with no lap swimming but eventually Dana did go to an indoor pool for a swim. That helped her some.

It was Tuesday, February 23, when Dana and Mike got a phone message after dinner.

Dana: My mother has fallen and can't get up.

Mike: We got over to their house and Dana helped her mother to a chair. I was alarmed. I got Dana off to the side and said that the left side of her face was drooping.

Dana: She's been having problems with her left knee. It's probably that and her face looks OK to me.

Mike: I went upstairs to check on Dana's father while Dana gave her mother a yogurt and then got her upstairs to a chair in the TV alcove next to their bedroom.

Dana's mother: I'm fine. I don't want to go the emergency room. Dana, you and Mike go home.

Dana: Maybe I should stay the night.

Dana's mother: No, I'll just go to bed. You go home.

Mike: Her voice was strong. She seemed completely in control as we were driving out Dana said.

Dana: Maybe I should stay.

Mike: She was definite. She did not want us there. We can come back if something happens.

Narrator: Mike and Dana drove home and figured that if anything happened, then her parents would call.

The call came the next morning. About 10 minutes before Anthony was due to arrive, Dana's father called. Her mother was on the floor. She had been on the floor all night.

Mike: Dana and I were stunned. All night? Why didn't someone call? Did Dana's mother say, "Guy, don't call Dana. Go to bed. Leave me alone." Did Dana's father really not realize until almost 7:00 then next morning that there was a problem? Did he just leave her on the floor?

Narrator: Dana went to her parents' house, got her mother an ambulance and to the ER. The stroke left her mother completely paralyzed on the left side and barely able to swallow. Dana mentioned the left knee problem to the neurologist who said, "Maybe so, but this is all from the stroke." Dana's mother was in an ICU bed and looked horrible. Since the Covid-19 protocols were in-place, only Dana could visit her mother. Her mother had not died, but over the next few days, it became apparent that she could barely talk or swallow. She would talk to Dana and seemed to know something of what had happened. She was stuck in a body that did not work and knew it. Mike thought this was a special kind of hell.

Mike: I still curse myself. The stroke was all my fault. I deferred to Dana and her parents, like I had always done. I should have ignored them and just called an ambulance. The fact that Dana's mother had a massive stroke is all my fault.

Narrator: Dana spent the night at her parents' house. The next day she arranged more people to come in and be with her father when Anthony was not there. Every day she and Mike would drive out to see her mother and check on her father. It was a lot of work and driving. Later in the week, she started looking for a place for her father live, some kind of assisted living.

Mike had friends, Ben and Suzanne Davis, who had used an assisted living facility called "The Forum at Memorial Woods." Dana called the Forum and a couple of other places. Only the Forum called her back. Early the next week, with Anthony's help, Dana's father was moved to a 2-bedroom apartment in the Forum.

Meanwhile, Dana's mother was able to swallow well enough to be transferred to a rehab hospital. She could not move anything on her left side. Standing or even sitting up was impossible. She could move her right hand well enough to drink something. She was drinking extraordinarily little and only taking in about 10% of the calories that the nurses thought she should be getting.

Mike: It took a few days to get Dana's father settled into a new location. Dana's father complained about the food. He said it was crap. This really rattled Dana. She questioned whether moving him was the right thing to do. I tried to argue that he could not stay in that house with a sequence of strangers taking care of him. As for the food, her mother had fought for years to try to find something he would like. She never succeeded.

Dana got a call from her primary saying that a blood test indicated a possible deep vein thrombosis. Her varicose veins had worsened over the last few years. She spent half a day at an ER and they found nothing. It just made for a long, and a little scary day.

It was all exhausting. Dana was not sleeping, and the anxiety was coming back. We managed to get a swim in that week, but I had to drive. Dana could not really go otherwise.

Dana: The anxiety is bad. My mind is out of control. I can't control my thoughts. I can't sleep. I am surrounded by old people. I am afraid that my life is over.

Mike: Do you want me to get you checked into a hospital?

Dana: They won't do it, besides what would they do?

Mike: They could just make you sleep.

Narrator: Dana called Psychiatrist-Mary and started back on Xanax. She filled a prescription for the "long lasting Xanax." She made an appointment for the following Tuesday with Psychiatrist-Mary. On Friday, she had a Zoom consultation with her principal care doctor about anxiety and depression. They went round and around trying to find an antidepressant that would not trigger a Long QT event. By the weekend, both Mike and Dana were exhausted.

It was Sunday morning and 4 days after Dana started back on Xanax.   Dana got up first, started a smoothy and made herself a coffee:

Dana: I'm in a very dark place.

Mike: I understand. Let me go and make some breakfast.

(Short time passes. Sound of a door slamming.)

Narrator: Mike went looking for Dana out the front door.

(Mannequin by a wall-corner with red shining all over the place. A cylinder by the left leg.)

Mike: Nooooo   not like this. Nooooo.

Narrator: Mike called 911. He was incoherent but eventually the operator said she'd send an ambulance. Mike went out the front gate. He paced, shivered, and cried. The ambulance came and he pointed inside the gate. He sat down next to a tree. Then the police came.

Police: Was she depressed? Did she know how to use a firearm?

Mike: Yes, she had been depressed and yes she knew how to shoot. We had done skeet shooting in the past.

I had to sign something for the ambulance guys acknowledging that they were not transporting anyone. A policeman asked me how long we had been married…. 37 years.

Narrator: Mike's neighbor, Gael Stack walked over with a friend David Ailsworth.

(Mike motions to them to stop and not come any closer. He walks over to them. He is shivering uncontrollably, unable to talk and crying.)

Gael Stack: Is it Dana?

(Mike nods.)

Gael Stack: Did she hurt herself?

(Mike nods and motions them to stay back. He is crying too much to talk.)

Narrator: More police arrive and then the medical examiner. One policeman walks across the street and rubs his shoes off in the grass. The policeman then went next door to tell the guys who lived there that something bad had happened. Gael and David stayed with Mike until everyone had left.

The medical examiner lead person was a young woman.

Medical examiner: We will bring her out in a few minutes. We had to bag her hands to check for gunpowder. We cleaned up as best we could, but you will need to get a professional cleaning service. Don't go over there.

Mike: Eventually, they rolled Dana out on a gurney. There was no mound for her head under the plastic. I watched her go. It didn't have to end this way. I should have stayed with her instead of making breakfast. It was only for a minute? This is all my fault.

Narrator: The police finished up and brought Mike a jacket to put on. He was still shivering and crying. The last policeman took away the gun. Eventually, he gave Mike his card and offered to talk. He drove away.

Mike: I managed to call my younger brother, Bill, in Kansas and asked him to tell my father in North Carolina. Bill said that he would fly down as soon as he could.

I went into the kitchen and threw out the uncooked eggs. Dana had started a smoothy but it only had one banana in it. We always put in one banana per person. Dana only put in one banana.

We had a cat, Clyde, who was a genuinely nice black cat. Clyde knew something bad had happened. I could not explain to him what, but he knew the world had changed.

Bill called and said that his wife, Karen, had arranged for him to arrive that night. It was Sunday morning still. I knew that I could not let him see where Dana had been. I went out to the garage and got a bucket, a broom and something to scrub with. I mixed up some detergent and got a hose.

I was still numb and not thinking straight at all. Have you ever cleaned up something like that? The blast blew parts of my wife over a ten-foot area. It took a long time to clean and rinse away parts of Dana. I cannot describe the horror. The medical examiner lady was probably right, but it was Sunday and how do you get something done on a Sunday during a pandemic?

The thought of it still makes me sick and sometimes sob. I threw away the clothes I was wearing. I threw away the broom, the scrubber, the bucket, and anything associated with that morning. There are foods that I cannot eat and TV shows that I can not watch. They bring back the images.

Later in the day, I called my father briefly and talked to a friend, Bob Woest, about how to tell Dana's parents. Bob is a practicing psychologist and had good advice.

That night, I made it to the airport to pick up Bill. I am certain that if he had not come down, I would not have lived through the week.

Bill: We got back to Mike's and Dana's house and I tried to get Mike to eat something. He couldn't eat more than a bite or two. His stomach was just sick or knotted up.   Then he tried to go to sleep.

Mike: That first night's sleep was hard. I couldn't get warm or stay asleep. The images kept coming back. I cursed myself for letting it happen. I could have done something. It was all my fault. The images kept coming back and back and still do.

Bill: It took a couple of days before Mike could eat a full plate of food. Even now, I ask him what he weighs. He needs to get on my diet to put weight back on.

The next day I went with Mike to tell Dana's father. Mike had made sure that his helper, Anthony, would be there. At first, Dana's father thought that Mike was talking about his wife dying. Then he understood but didn't react much.

When Mike went to tell Dana's mother, I had to wait in the car, because of the Covid-19 pandemic rules. Mike came back and said that Dana's mother didn't really say anything, but he thought that he saw a tear in one eye.

As the week went on, I went with Mike to the funeral parlor to make arrangements for Dana. The guy at the funeral home wanted a picture to use to identify Dana. Mike said it wouldn't do him any good. He did not ask any more questions. Later in the week, we picked up Dana's father and Anthony, drove to the cemetery and placed Dana's ashes next to her brother's. Mike had picked out a reading and asked me to read it, Micah 6:8:
> "You have been told, O mortal, what is good, and what the
> Lord requires of you
> Only to do justice and to love goodness and to walk
> humbly with your God."

Mike couldn't read it. He was way too choked up. I barely got it out.

I helped him with some errands, like turning in a leased Lexus. My wife, Karen, who is a veterinarian, talked to Mike's cat vet and arranged for Mike to turn over Clyde. Dana and Mike had raised Clyde from a rescue kitten, 6 years earlier, but Mike couldn't take care of him. It was hard for Mike to give Clyde away, but we later learned that they had found him a new home within a day. Clyde was in a new caring home, but it was not easy. I went home to Kansas the next weekend. By the time I left, Mike could at least eat a little better.

Mike: Bill's trip saved my life. There is no way I could have made it through the week without him being there. It took a few days to be able to eat and two of my neighbors brought over food. The food helped. Bill still asks me how much weight I've lost. I think I was probably 16 the last time I weighed this much. It is still hard to eat, and some foods just remind me of Dana, of our life together or of what I saw that morning.

Neither of Dana's parents every asked what happened to Dana and I never told them. I only said that "she died." It's as if they somehow knew. I know that when she was a teenager, there were "problems" and she had seen a therapist. Dana had talked about that time, but it was never really explained me. Her parents had seen her years before during "the Troubles" and knew that she was struggling then. Did her parents just know?

Narrator: During the next couple of weeks, Mike had to write Dana's obituary and order a headstone, with an added line, "She was a light to us all."

There were bills to pay and lots of details to chase down. Also, Mike had a designated power of attorney for both of Dana's parents, but companies had to be notified. Mike has always hated this kind of work, but he realized that for a while this would be his new "job."

Dana's father needed almost daily support. He needed to get a Covid shot, go to the doctor, get prescriptions, and get settled into his assisted living apartment. There were lots of trips to Dana's parents' house to pick up stuff and check mail. Anthony had agreed to continue working with Dana's father, just in a different environment. Anthony Martin was essential.

In the meantime, Dana's mother was making no progress in recovering from the stroke. She was only eating 10-20% of what she would need to consume to maintain weight. The rehab hospital said that Medicare would not let them keep her if she was making no "measurable progress." She was not and eventually the rehab people shipped her to the Forum. She was in the same building as Dana's father, but on a different floor, in "Skilled Nursing." She would talk with the nursing staff some and drink some, but still made little or no progress.

Dana was part of an extended Facebook community and her loss affected lots of people. Mike was able to use her Facebook account to put out a message. People started sending Mike condolences which helped...A lifeguard at the pool, Nadine, brought by a pool and arranged for the lap swimming crowd to sign a card. Mike cried when he read the card. Mike's nephew, Michael, who was a first-year medical student, wrote a long letter that Mike could barely read through the tears.   All of the letters, emails, texts and cards brought on more tears. They still do.

A couple of weeks after Bill left, Mike's father and older brother came, picked him up and they all drove to Kansas to Bill's house. The visit helped Mike get through another week. Mike, his brother and father then drove to the family home in Charlotte, N.C. They drove up to the mountains to visit Mike's cousin Catherine and her family. She made lunch and let them feel normal for a couple of hours. Some family friends, the Fespermans, brought over lunch. It helped Mike to see them. They knew pain and loss. Mike is still deeply moved by all of the kindness that people have showed. The kindnesses help him through his waking hours.

Mike still wakes up in the middle of the night and sees the images. He knows that those images will always be there. Night and trying to sleep are always the worst times.

Mike: Jim Meehan, a friend who lost his wife several years ago to cancer, sent me a long letter about "the Void." He talked about the Void always being in you and with you. Mine seems to be partially filled with sadness, with guilt and with a sick feeling that will not go away.

I have started the think that the Void comes from a heart-shattering event. A heart-breaking event is something like a broken arm. It leaves a scar but otherwise heals up and life goes on. A heart-shattering event is like throwing a glass against the floor and then trying to glue it back together. Some pieces may fit back, but there are always pieces that get lost or don't fit. They leave voids in what you have tried to put back together. Dana's loss was or is a heart-shattering event for me. It has left a void that sits right in the front of my chest. It's like a piece of my beating heart is missing. Jim is right about the Void.

Narrator: Anthony was able to arrange a way for Dana's father to see and visit with Dana's mother. Because of all of the Covid-19 restrictions, the first meeting had to take place in an open patio. Dana's mother was wheeled in on a reclining sort of chair-bed. Anthony wheeled in Dana's father in his wheelchair.

Mike: Talking to Anthony later, I found out that Dana's mother would not respond to or answer a question from Dana's father. She just lay on her chair and waited for the time to go by. Anthony found out that before going down there, Dana's mother had been talking to the nurses, but when she got back to her room, she was angry and agitated.

Anthony and Dana's father tried one more meeting, but it was the same. Dana's mother would not talk to him. For that matter, she would not talk to me anymore either. She did not want to see either of us.

Dana's mother only said one thing to me. After I told her that Dana had died, she said, "We'll keep going." Dana's father said almost the exact same thing to me. The two of them would keep going, even though, now, both of their children were dead.

Narrator: On a Tuesday morning, Mike took some supplies to Dana's father and headed back home. Before he could get home, Anthony called to say that Dana's father had filled up a diaper with a black tarry mess. Mike needed to come back immediately.

Mike: I was in the car driving so, I pulled off into a parking lot and called the front desk of the Forum. The receptionist said she could call an ambulance. I headed back but missed the ambulance and headed west on I-10 to the most likely ER, at the Memorial-Hermann hospital on Gessner. It was hours before I could see Dana's father. By then, they had started tests and had given him a unit of blood.

Over the next day or 2, tests were run, and I talked to the gastroenterologist that he had seen him a few years earlier. He made the case that the pre-cancerous polyps that they had been seen before had now evolved into full stomach cancer. The stomach cancer was not operable because of his heart. It made no sense to even do endoscopy. Seeing something or knowing more would not change the clinical outcome.

Anthony visited Dana's father in the hospital and kept him company on Friday of that week while I started the hospice enrollment procedures. The first step was a conference call with the hospital's "End of Life" care team. I was in the room with them while on the line were Dana's cousin and her husband, Paige and Paul, in Baton Rouge. Paige and Paul have had long careers as physical therapists. They knew the right questions to ask. We were all impressed at how competently the hospital's team operated. They did a superb job of managing a gut-wrenching situation.

Paige and Paul had already helped me order a special wheelchair for Dana's mother. Paige was Dana's only remaining cousin on her mother's side. They had 2 daughters and a son that we had watched grow up. The whole family is a set of solid, good people. Their help with Dana's parents was a huge thing for me.

Later that Friday, I signed the paperwork for hospice. The plan was to move him back to his apartment at the Forum and start hospice there. In the hospital, they had ceased transfusions, tests and unplugged his IV. Before I left, Dana's father said, "Be careful on the freeway with the rain." I then headed back to the Forum to check on Dana's mother and then home.

Narrator: The phone call came at about 6:55 pm. Dana's father had died. Mike was shocked. Dana's father had seemed strong at 2:00 pm.

Mike: None of us had any idea that he had such advanced stomach cancer. He had seen his regular internist about 3 weeks earlier and was scheduled for a follow-up in 6 months. One of the things that drove Dana's anxiety was the idea of having to take care of an invalid father and mother for years into the future. It makes me crazy. I cannot think about this.

Narrator: The sequence started all over again. Mike asked Theresa Frierson, the attorney who had handled Dana's will to handle Dana's father's will. He called Tripp Carter at BradshawCarter. Tripp remembered Mike from working with Dana, 5 weeks earlier. The next day Mike went in and made the arrangements and later found the "urn" that had been purchased through the Neptune Society. Tripp made the arrangements with Glenwood Cemetery.

Mike told Dana's mother that her husband had died and about the cancer. He thought that he saw a tear in her eye, but otherwise she made no response and said nothing. The next day Anthony visited Dana's mother and re-told her about her husband. She seemed to respond a little to Anthony, but really, very little.

Mike: My car was in the shop, so I had to ride my bike to the cemetery the morning of the internment. I had told Tripp that I did not want any chairs or special stuff. They had put down some grass-colored carpet that covered Dana's ashes. I moved it back.

Tripp helped me with a reading: Zechariah, 8:16-17:
>"These then are the things you must do:
>Speak the truth to one another, judge with honesty and
>complete justice at your gates.
>Let none of you plot evil against another in your heart, nor
>love a false oath.
>For all these things I hate – oracle of the Lord."

We said a Lord's prayer, closed the crypt for his ashes and Dylan
from Glenwood lowered everything down.

Dylan Carroll was the manager for the grounds at Glenwood. He
remembered me from Dana's ash-placing a not many weeks
earlier. We talked about trees and placing some around. We talked
about bicycling along the bayou. Eventually, a crew came and
filled in the hole. I said a few more prayers and rode my bike
home, the long way.

Narrator: Over the next 2 weeks, Dana's mother's condition
deteriorated. Mike would later learn from the nurse that a change
for the worse started as soon as she heard about her husband.
Dana's mother, like her father, had signed a document declining
any sort of invasive care to extend her life, including extra-
hydration. Since she was still drinking a tiny amount, her urinary
output diminished, and her blood chemistry started to show signs
of real dehydration. With Paige and Paul's help, a decision was
made to move to hospice. A hospice group, Crossroads, that the
Forum had lots of experience with had staff on-site the day Mike
signed the paperwork.

Mike: I started riding my bike from home to the Forum. It took
about 45 minutes one way on my hard-tail mountain bike. Most of
the way was on paved bike paths but there was a little off-road
now and then. I took small things in my backpack, like pictures
which Dana's mother might recognize. It was never clear if she
recognized any of the pictures on the table by her bed. She never

spoke to me. At this point, she was on morphine and other things "to make her comfortable." She just never spoke again or even nodded.

On the second or third day, one of the Crossroads hospice nurses stopped in at the same time that I was there. Her name was Dawn and I had spoken with her on the phone once before. With Covid-19 protocols in-place, she kept her mask on and was in full-blue nurse's pant-suit uniform. She carefully checked over Dana's mother and showed real kindness. We talked a little and I tried to explain some of the pictures and a little about Dana's mother and father. I was trying to humanize this end life process. She finished and I stayed a while longer. She was doing a job that I could not do, and I said so.

Dawn-hospice: It is a privilege to work with people like Mrs. Birmingham in this part of their life.

Mike: Dawn and the Forum nurses said that Dana's mother could hear us. So, I would try to talk when we were alone. Even though she was totally non-religious, like the rest of the family, I would pray and read Psalms or other verses. If she understood what I was doing, I am certain it would have annoyed her. One verse that I read several times, because I thought it applied to both of us, was from the book of Judith before Judith went off to kill Holofernes, Judith 9:11: "Your strength is not in numbers, nor does your might depend upon the powerful.
   You are God of the lowly, helper of those of little account, supporter of the weak, protector of those in despair, savior of those without hope."

If she could understand what I was reading, I think she might understand why Judith's prayer applied to both of us.

Years ago, I had read a book about death and dying from the Buddhist point of view. It talked about going toward the light and a sound of crickets that could help guide you. I told Dana's mother to follow the sound of the crickets and to go toward the light. I told her that it was OK to go. Dawn later asked me if I had given Dana's mother permission to go. I said, "Yes." We both thought she was holding on, but Dawn thought she was at peace.

Dawn-hospice: Sometimes you can go in a room and tell that someone is fighting it, that they are not at peace. She is at peace, but she is still holding on.

Mike: On a later day, Dawn and I overlapped again. I had brought a picture of Dana's mother as an 18-year-old in a long pink formal gown. I thought that perhaps Dana's mother could recognize herself from an earlier time and remember better days. Dana's mother had been a strikingly beautiful young woman in the early 1950's.

Dawn really like the pink dress and I said I'd give it to her if it turned up among their things. I sure did not want it. We talked about where Dana's parents had lived and traveled to, and she mentioned she was a salt-water girl.

About that time, she went over to the door, shut it, came back, and took off her mask. I knew from the ID picture on her badge that she was both young and exceptionally good looking. With our masks off, we talked about her living in Brazil, where her husband was from, about islands, surfing and not liking the cold. She talked about the Caymans and that her family normally went there once a year, the last time just before the Covid-19 lockdown. It made me actually want to go to the Caymans. It is a set of islands that Dana and I never visited.

I know that the hospice people are there to help family members also. She was doing her job. Still, her kindness and gentleness were jarring in a seismic way to an old man like me who lived in an emotional fog. She allowed me to have a moment of what felt like normal, easy conversation. It was a brief glimpse of life away from everything I was living.

Narrator: When Mike arrived on about the seventh day of hospice, Dana's mother looked worse than the day before. She did not move her head or even seem to see the pictures on the table by the bed. Her breathing consisted of 6 to 7 short breaths followed by a long period of no breathing, apnea.

Mike: I texted Dawn: "I may be mistaken but I think Mrs. Birmingham has settled into a Cheyne-Stokes breathing pattern. Apnea seems to be 21-23 seconds."

Dawn texted back: "Oh my. Ok. I'll be down shortly."

When she arrived, I asked, "How much longer?"

Dawn-hospice: The erratic breathing is causing the CO_2 level in her blood to rise. Eventually, it will trigger a cardiac event.

Mike: So, 6-12 hours?

Dawn-hospice: At most, probably more like 4-5.

Narrator: Dawn stayed a few more minutes and then Mike rode his bike home to clean up. He returned about an hour and a half later. He would never encounter Dawn again. He knew that she saw many elderly family members like him every week, but still her kindness had been a glimmer of light.

Mike: I spent the afternoon sitting with Dana's mother. She was consistently in a Cheyne-Stokes breathing pattern. There would be 6-7 gasping breaths and then 21-29 seconds of apnea, no breathing. I prayed and read some scripture to her. I told her to follow the crickets and go toward the light. I told her it was OK to go. Because of all of the morphine, I doubt she heard anything I said.

She was completely non-responsive, but it was an attempt to let her know that she was not alone.

At about 4:46 pm, Dana's mother took 2 breaths and made a grimaced look of pain with each. All of the color drained out of her face, down to a stony white. She did not take another breath.

I went down the hall and got the nurse. She came back and verified that there was no pulse. I knelt down and said a final prayer, picked up the personal things and went home. I was sick to my stomach.

Narrator: The sequence started all over again. Mike asked Theresa Frierson, the attorney, to handle another will. Mike called Tripp Carter at BradshawCarter. Tripp was sorry to hear from Mike so soon. He would be out with a surgery so someone else would work this through. The next day Mike went in and made the arrangements and delivered the "urn" that had been purchased through the Neptune Society. More arrangements were made at Glenwood Cemetery for a private and simple internment. Dylan Carroll called to say that he was sorry to hear from Mike so soon and offered a discount since it would be another small event.

Mike called Paige and Paul in Baton Rouge. He also made another call to Dana's father's sister in Midland, Mary Cohlmia. This was now the third call to Mrs. Cohlmia to tell her about a death in the family. For everyone on both sides of the family, the loss was now complete, Britton, Dana, mother, and father.

Mike: For the internment of Dana's mother's ashes, I rode my bike again. It seemed reasonable for a family revolved around bike riding on so many occasions. I was not in control so the rep from BradshawCarter read for me the same reading that was used for Britton and Dana: Micah 6:8:
> "You have been told, O mortal, what is good, and what the
> Lord requires of you,

Only to do justice and to love goodness and to walk humbly with your God."

We said a Lord's Prayer and then waited. Like I had done with Dana and her father, I placed some things and a few pictures with the ashes. Dylan Carroll from Glenwood came over and lowered the crypt into the ground. Then we waited, and I knelt down on the green carpet again.

An older man, my age, that I had seen visiting the graves next to Dana's family saw me kneeling and praying. He came over and took off his shoes at the edge of the green carpet. He knelt down, put a cell phone on the carpet and began to pray. The cell phone was playing a dirge in Arabic. It was a slow and very sorrowful prayer sung by a single voice.

As he prayed, I prayed as well. In a few minutes, he stopped praying and came over to shake my hand and explain that he had seen me before placing flowers and praying. He said that his parents and brother were all nearby. He said that Dana and her family were in heaven. I was totally choked up and tried to say something, or just thanks.

He had made the Sign-of-the-Cross and confirmed that the dirge was in Arabic. The Middle East does have some Christians. I have not seen him at Glenwood since that day but hope to see him again. He did a kind thing, praying with me.

As we waited for the grounds crew, I talked with Dylan about trees, and we made small talk. They picked up the carpet, picked up the lowering machine and filled in the hole. I rode my bike home.

Narrator: Mike goes back periodically to change out cut flowers. Britton's grave marker has been at Glenwood since 2015. While waiting on four more grave markers, Mike made up some temporary ones using laminating sheets and wooden stakes he made in the garage. With Covid-19, it takes months to get grave markers made. Dana's headstone should be ready before the other 3. Mike has not seen the man with the Arabic dirge since the placing of those last ashes.

Mike is still not thinking clearly.

Mike: I cannot get my mind around any of this. Part of it may be the void, the sadness, and the fog of it all. In Job's final reply, he says: (Job 31: 5:15):

> "If I have walked in falsehood and my foot has hastened to deceit,
> Let God weigh me in the scales of justice; thus, will he know my innocence!
> If my steps have turned out of the way, and my heart has followed my eyes, or any stain clings to my hands,
> Then may I sow, but another eat, and may my produce be rooted up!
> If my heart has been enticed toward a woman, and I have lain in wait at my neighbor's door;
> Then may my wife grind for another, and may others kneel over her! 11For that would be heinous, a crime to be condemned.
> A fire that would consume down to Abaddon till it uprooted all my crops.
> Had I refused justice to my manservant or to my maidservant, when they had a complaint against me,
> What then should I do when God rises up? What could I answer when he demands an account?
> Did not he who made me in the belly make him? Did not the same One fashion us in the womb?"

Job must have been a young man. He can argue for his innocence, but I would never. When Jesus said that whoever is without sin should cast the first stone, Job could throw, but I could never. It is interesting how much Job focuses on himself. All of his kids are killed but he looks at his own suffering. Did he ever feel the Void?

Nothing that Job ever said or did was of any relevance to what happened to him. Job did not know that it was God who gave the devil free reign to torture him. God never explained this to Job, but he did show himself to Job. At the end, Job could conclude: (Job 42:5-6):
"By hearsay I had heard of you, but now my eye has seen you. Therefore, I disown what I have said, and repent in dust and ashes."

Nothing with Dana makes any sense. In physics you learn that some things can not be known. The Heisenberg Uncertainty Principle says that you cannot simultaneously know both position and momentum exactly. If you know one exactly, the other is completely indeterminate. If two star-systems are separated by a distance farther than light could have traveled in the history of the universe, one cannot know about the other… until sometime in the future. Are the reasons for Dana's death simply unknowable or are they simply my fault? The truth is staring me in the face, making me sick.

The sick truth of it all is that even if I had every answer to every question, Dana would still be gone …. nothing would fundamentally change.

Narrator: Mike is still waiting for the estates of Dana's parents to go through probate. All of their assets go in equal amounts to 3 charities. Mike will likely be appointed executor and must get everything sold, proceeds delivered and then handle final tax filings next year. It will take a while. This is why Mike is in Dana's parents' kitchen waiting for some estate brokers.

(Mike sits in a chair and then turns toward the audience.)

Mike: You must be wondering why I would try to tell a story like this. If I had acted differently, at least, Dana and her mother would still be alive. This horrible tragedy is my fault.

One reason to tell this story is that throughout the last few months, many people have been truly kind to me. Whether it was friends who talked on the phone, those who sent messages, brought food, or people who helped me directly, like the middle eastern man with his Arabic dirge, these people have been kind to me, and I want them to know how grateful I am. Really, for this whole ten years, many people have been far more generous, and kind to me than I deserve.

A week or so ago, there was a thing in the news about a young woman, a professional athlete, with anxiety and depression. She had to drop out of a tournament. I wondered if, like Dana, she would be told, "You're so strong. There can't be anything wrong with you." I quietly hoped that young woman would have the physical sources of her depression and anxiety ruled out before starting down the psychiatry-drug-addiction trail. Is that young woman already doped up?

How many people will be prescribed Prozac or one of the other Long QT drugs and then be found dead in their bedroom?

How many people will call or visit an ER, describe agonal breathing and fixed-eye stare and be told it's probably the flu or menstrual problems?

If any part of this story resonates with you, please do a better job than I did.

Neither Dana nor anyone in her family was religious but after each of their deaths, I've asked Paul English or Joseph Pilsner or another Basilian priest to remember them at Mass.

I know that Dana did not believe in any of this, but it is the only hope that I have. If Dana was right and after this life there is nothingness, then I am OK with that. For me it would mean that the images would stop.

I admit that I do not know which version of the afterlife is correct. I don't think that I have faith or a real belief in any specific scenario, only hope. I hope that there is a heaven, and that Dana is in it, along with her family and many others.

(Kneel)
"Lord God, please may Dana be with you in Paradise.
This, my Lord God, I ask through the name of your Son, Jesus Christ."
(Touch head to the ground 3 times.)
Say the Lord's Prayer.

(Stay kneeling)

If Dana is in heaven, then that is where I want to be.
If Dana is in hell, then that is where I want to be.
If the cost of Dana being in heaven is me in hell, then send me to hell.

(Mike gets up.)

Mike: Thank you for listening to Dana's story. I know that parts are hard to understand, and I don't understand what has happened these last 3 months. I am still in a fog of sadness for Dana. When I think of joining her, I get the most pleasant sense of calm, of peace.

A couple of weeks ago on television, the network was re-showing the movie, "Gladiator." I switched on the TV to a scene where the former general, now a gladiator-slave, is sitting on a parapet with another gladiator-slave, a young black African. They talk about the next life and family waiting for them there. The general says that his wife and son are already waiting for him there. The young African says that he will see them, "Just not yet." I turned off the TV. I understood their desire to see their loved ones in the next life and I understood that for whatever reason, for me, it is still, "Just not yet."

(Turn off all lights.)
(Female voice singing "Amazing Grace" with a single guitar as accompaniment.)

Author's notes:

1. All of the Bible quotes in this piece are from the "Saint Benedict Press, New American Bible, Revised Edition," 2011, ISBN: 978-1,-935302-57-5, Saint Benedict Press, LLC, Charlotte, NC, USA.
2. Good discussions of thyroid function can be found in:
    a. Kovacs, William J. and Ojeda, Sergio R., "Textbook of Endocrine Physiology, Sixth Edition," Oxford University Press, 2012.
    b. Tortora, Gerard J. and Grabowski, I., "Principles of Anatomy and Physiology, Eight Edition," Biological Sciences Textbooks, 1996.
3. Author's request, if you have found this story at all interesting or relevant:
    a. Please share a copy of this with someone who you think might benefit from it.
    b. Please donate to the "Dana K. Padgett Excellence in Art Graduate Scholarship Endowment" at the University of Houston. It is a scholarship fund for art graduate students, both studio and art history, at U of H. Your donation will help students pursue their careers in art…......
    c. Thank you.

Supplemental material:

Plot of TSH vs Free-T4 after the treatments by Arem had started to work.

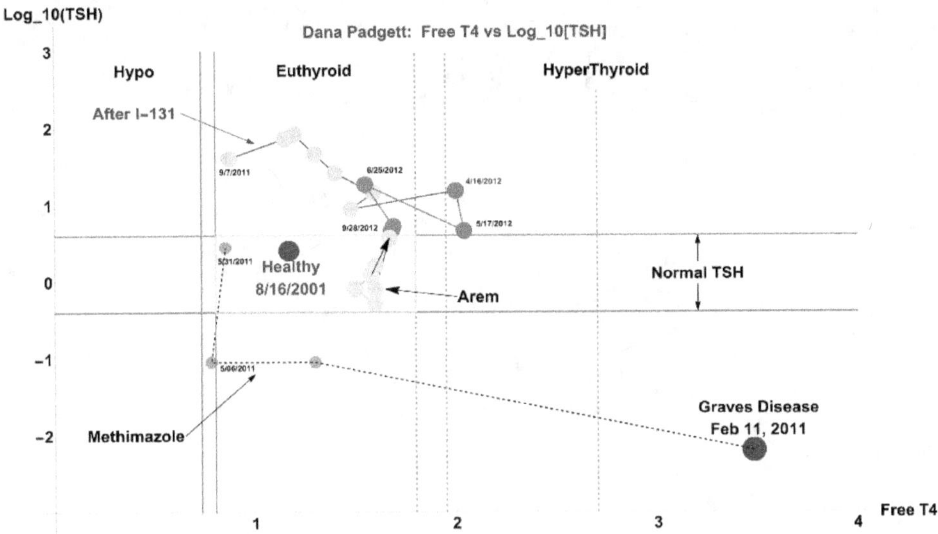

EKG strips on 9-6-2015

starting at 13:48

PADGETT,DANA 8634 06-Sep-2015 13:48:25
HR 46 PVC 0 ST II 0.7
TTX# 8634AP

TELE|504*TTX# 8634AP

25 mm/s

PADGETT,DANA 8634 06-Sep-2015 13:48:31

V TACH HR 105 PVC 0 ST II 0.7

TTX# 8634AP

V TACH

25 mm/s

PADGETT,DANA 8634 06-Sep-2015 13:48:36

TELE|504*TTX# 8634AP

V TACH HR 101 PVC 8 ST II 0.7 Alarms Silenced
TTX# 8634AP

V TACH

PVC

II
(0.1)

III
(-0.2)

VT
(0.4)

aVR
(0.6)

aVL
(0.5)

aVF
(0.1)

25 mm/s

PADGETT,DANA 8634 06-Sep-2015 14:06:08

TELE|504*TTX# 8634AP

PVC HR 50 PVC 0 ST I 0.4
TTX# 8634AP

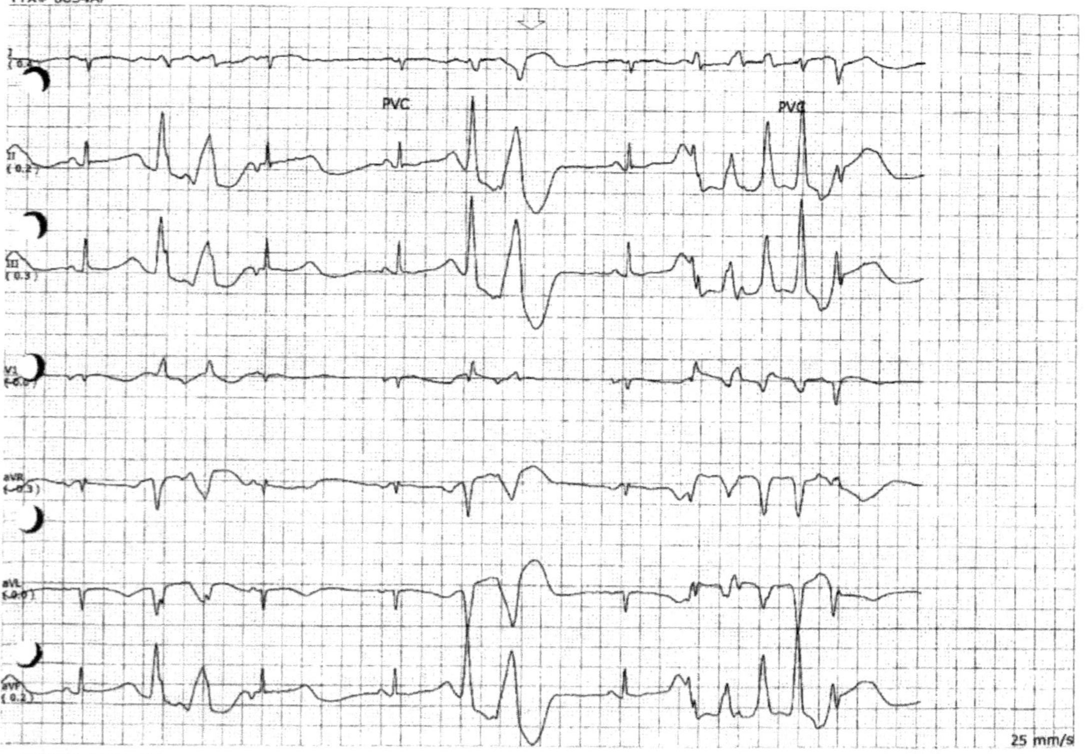

PADGETT,DANA 8634 06-Sep-2015 14:06:12   TELE|504*TTX# 8634AP
PVC HR 59 PVC 1 ST I 0.4
TTX# 8634AP

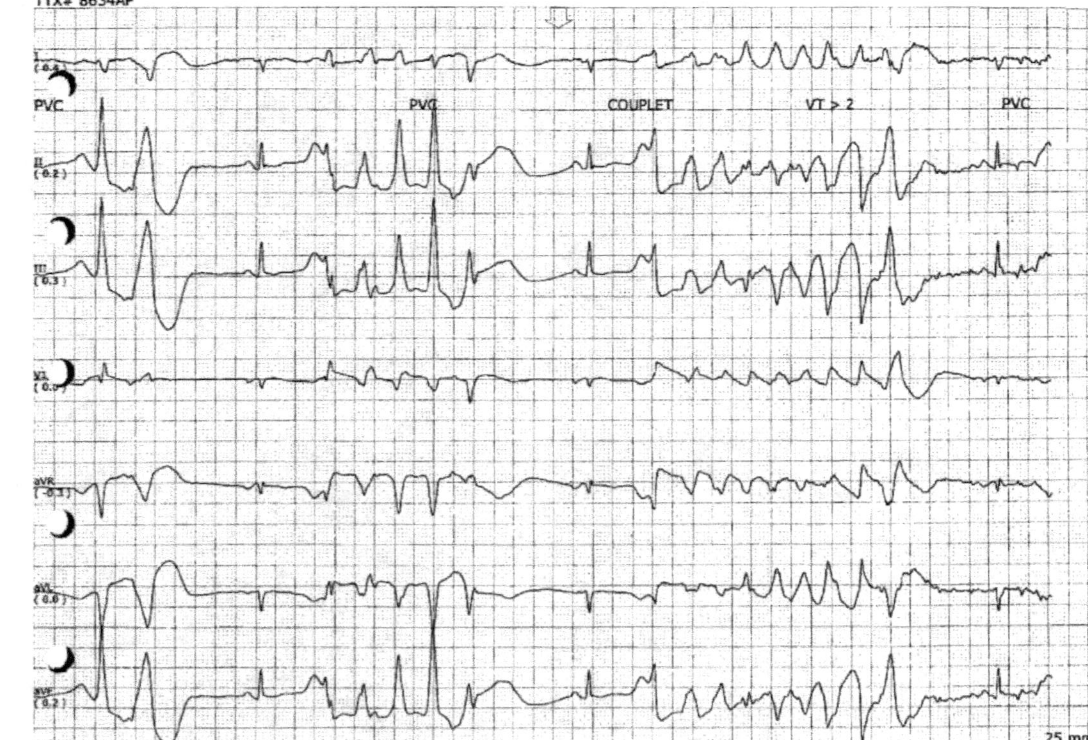

PADGETT,DANA 8634 06-Sep-2015 14:06:12

TELE|504*TTX# 8634AP

PVC HR 59 PVC 1 ST I 0.4

TTX# 8634AP

PVC

PVC

COUPLET

VT > 2

PVC

II
(0.2)

III
(0.3)

V1
(0.0)

aVR
(-0.3)

aVL
(0.0)

aVF
(0.2)

25 mm/s

PADGETT,DANA 8634 06-Sep-2015 14:06:33

TELE|504*TTX# 8634AP

TRIGEMINY HR 68 PVC 22 ST II 0.5

TTX# 8634AP

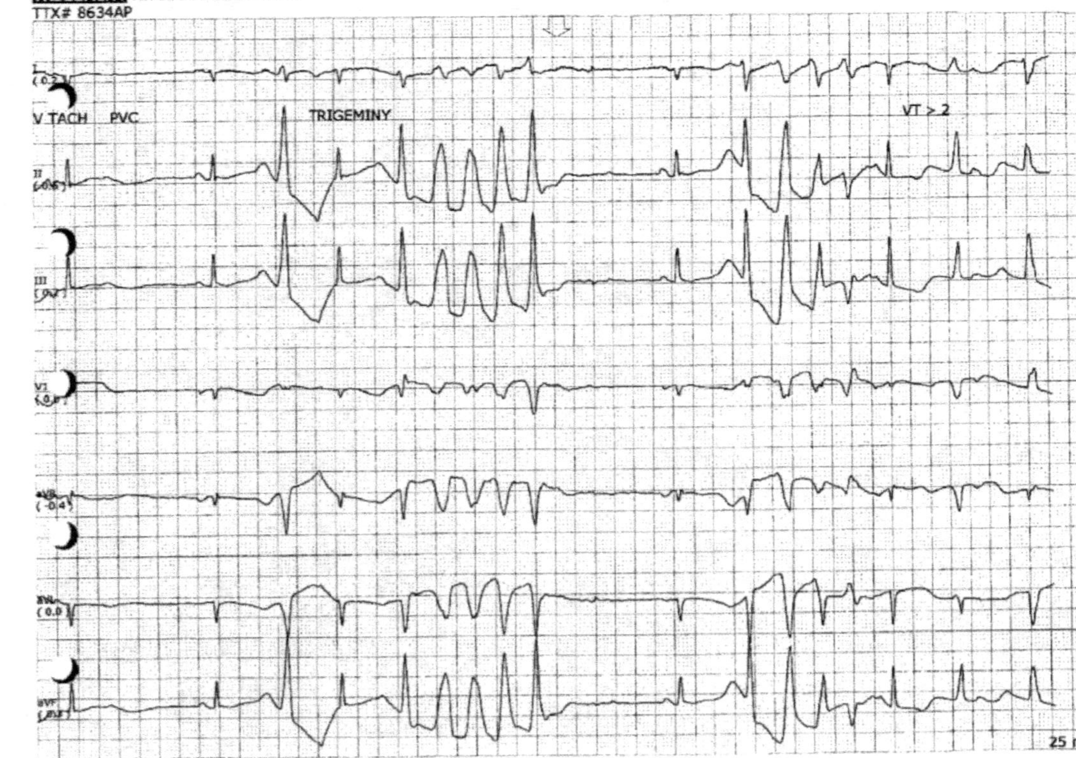

CARESCAPE Central Station V1 (6.0.6).
Sunday, September 06, 2015 2:08:05 PM

Page 1
END OF REPORT

PADGETT,DANA 8634 06-Sep-2015 14:06:37

TELE|504*TTX# 8634AP

VT > 2 HR 89 PVC 24 ST II 0.5

TTX# 8634AP

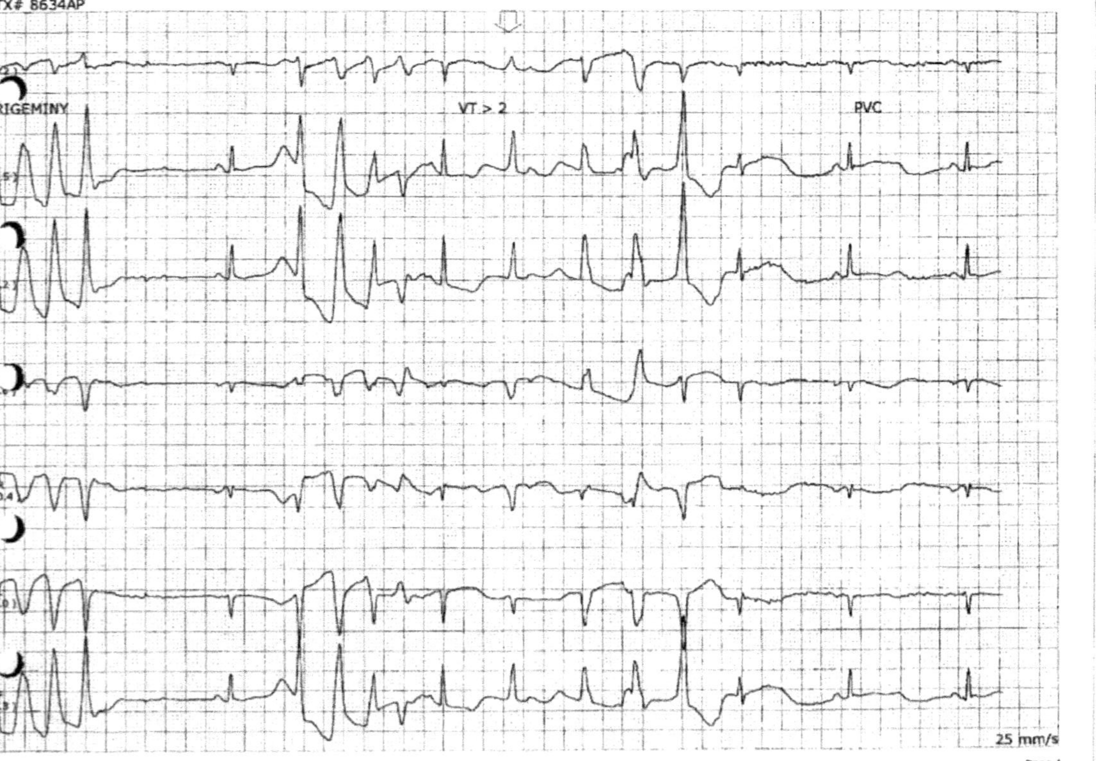

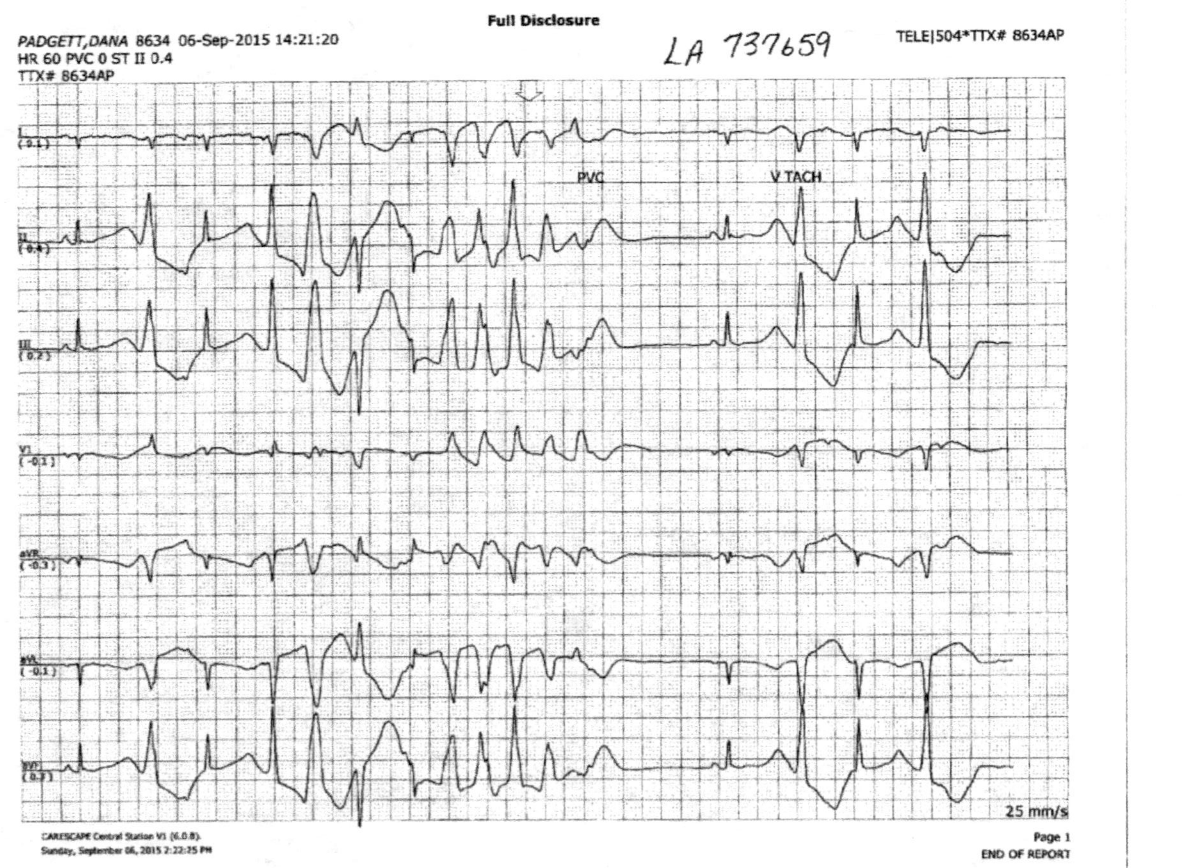

Full Disclosure
PADGETT,DANA 8634 06-Sep-2015 14:21:20
HR 60 PVC 0 ST II 0.4
TTX# 8634AP
LA 737659
TELE|504*TTX# 8634AP
I (0.1)
II (0.4)
III (0.2)
V1 (-0.1)
aVR (-0.3)
aVL (-0.1)
aVF (0.3)
PVC
V TACH
25 mm/s
CARESCAPE Central Station V1 (6.0.8).
Sunday, September 06, 2015 2:22:35 PM
Page 1
END OF REPORT

PADGETT,DANA 8634 06-Sep-2015 14:12:25   TELE|504*TTX# 8634AP

PVC HR 94 PVC 11 ST II 0.3 Alarms Silenced

TTX# 8634AP

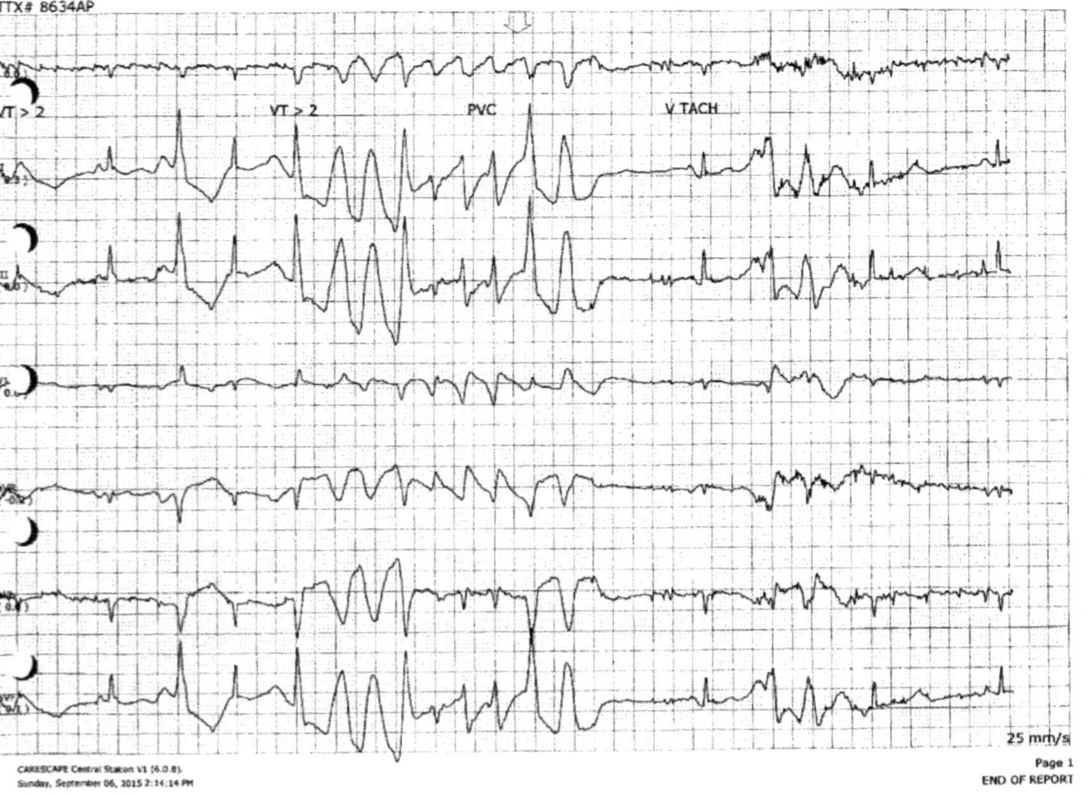

PADGETT,DANA 8634 06-Sep-2015 14:27:22

COUPLET HR 63 PVC 3 ST II 0.8

TTX# 8634AP

TELE|504*TTX# 8634AP

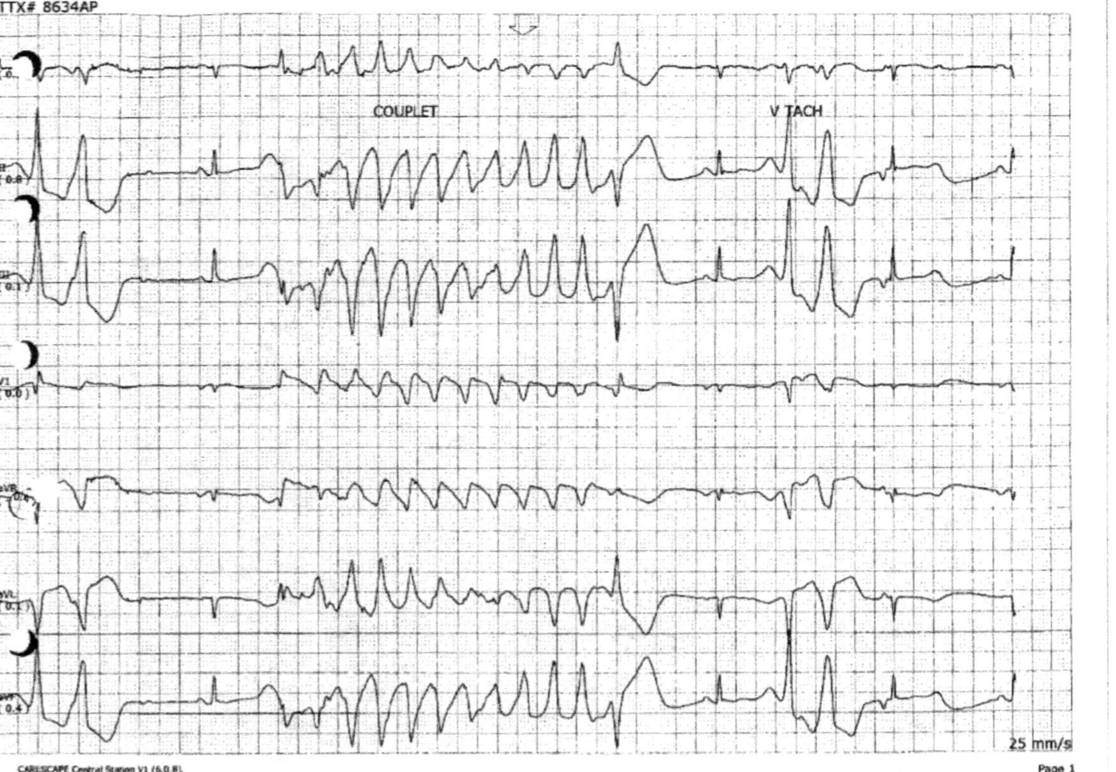

EKG strips on 9-6-2015

starting at 14:55

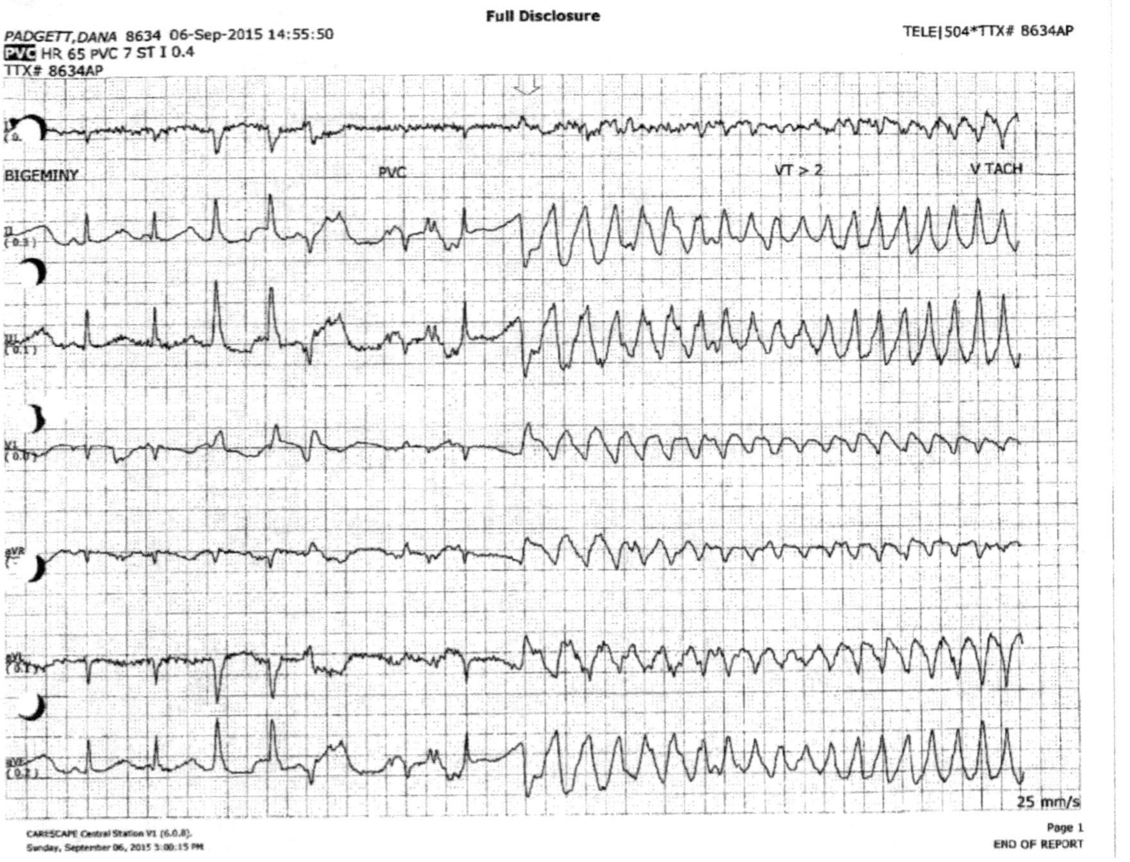
Full Disclosure
PADGETT,DANA 8634 06-Sep-2015 14:55:50
TELE|504*TTX# 8634AP
PVC HR 65 PVC 7 ST I 0.4
TTX# 8634AP
BIGEMINY
PVC
VT > 2
V TACH
25 mm/s
CARESCAPE Central Station V1 (6.0.8).
Sunday, September 06, 2015 5:00:15 PM
Page 1
END OF REPORT

PADGETT,DANA 8634 06-Sep-2015 14:55:58

TELE|504*TTX# 8634AP

VFIB/VTAC HR 0 PVC 16 ST I 0.4

TTX# 8634AP

VT > 2   V TACH   VFIB/VTAC   V TACH

25 mm/s

PADGETT,DANA 8634 06-Sep-2015 14:56:16
TELE|504*TTX# 8634AP
V TACH HR 183 PVC 53 ST I 0.4
TTX# 8634AP

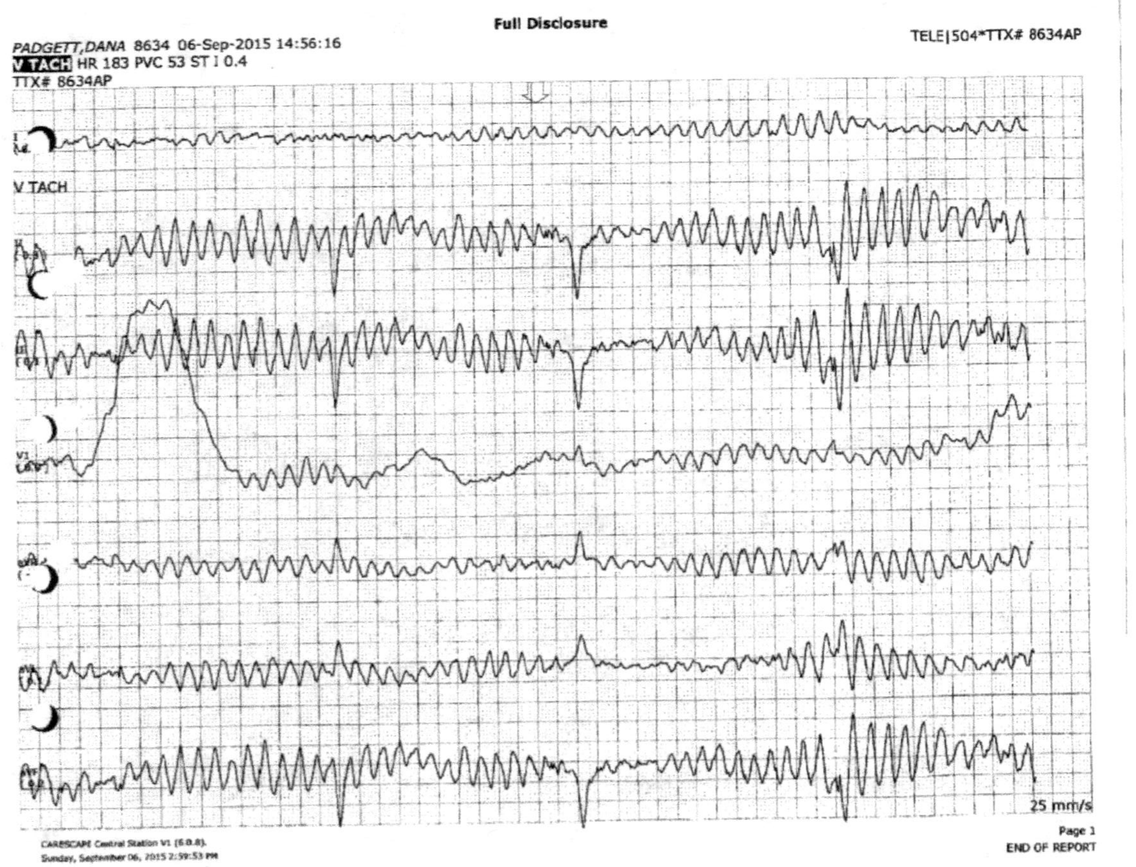

CARESCAPE Central Station V1 (6.0.8).
Sunday, September 06, 2015 2:59:53 PM

PADGETT,DANA 8634 06-Sep-2015 14:56:30

TELE|504*TTX# 8634AP

V TACH HR 0 PVC 71 ST II X

TTX# 8634AP

VFIB/VTAC   V TACH

25 mm/s

CARESCAPE Central Station V1 (6.0.6).
Sunday, September 06, 2015 2:59:29 PM

Page 1
END OF REPORT

I (X)

III (X)

R (X)

aVF (X)

V (X)

I (X)

II (X)

III (X)

AVR (X)

(X)

AVF (X)

V (X)

I (X)

II (X)

III (X)

AVR (X)

(X)

AVF (X)

IV (X)

I (X)

II (X)

III (X)

AVR (X)

(X)

AVF (X)

V (X)

PADGETT,DANA 8634 06-Sep-2015 14:58:55

TELE|504*TTX# 8634AP

HR 69 PVC 86 ST I 0.4

TTX# 8634AP

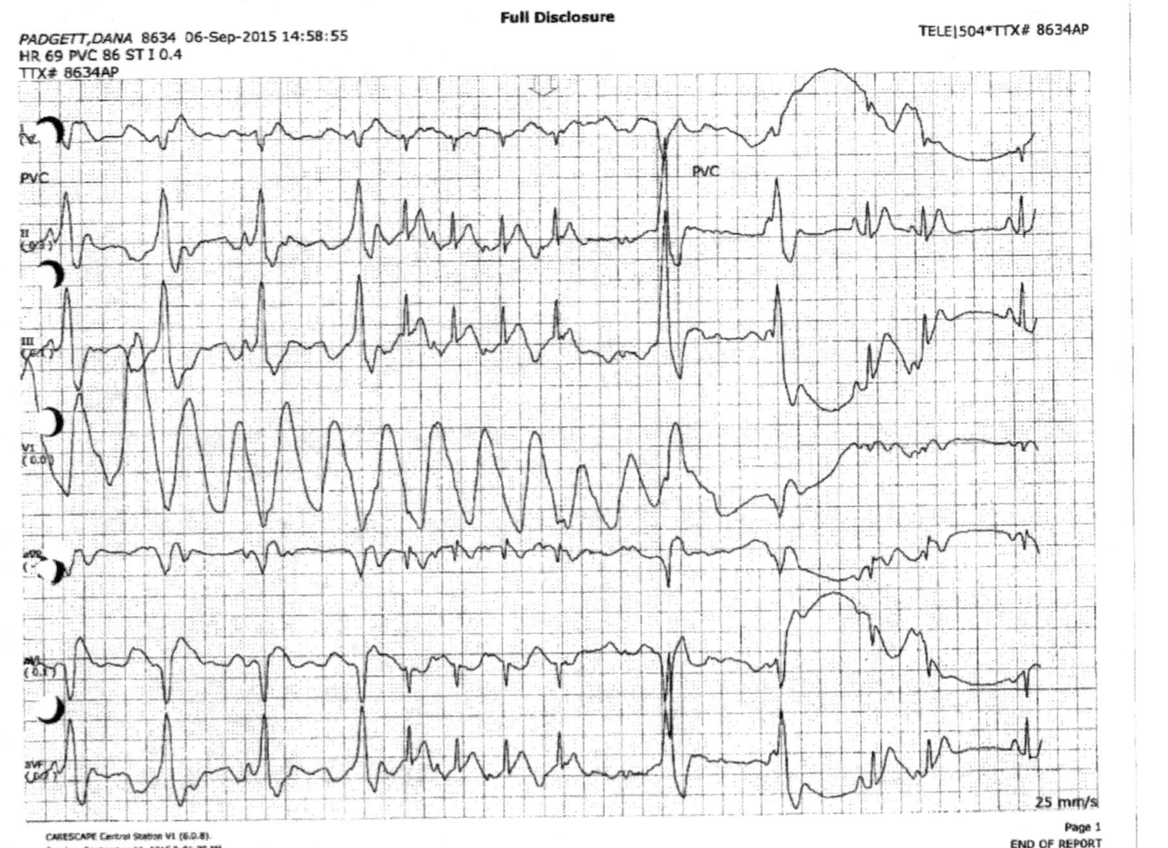

Pictures from travel and life

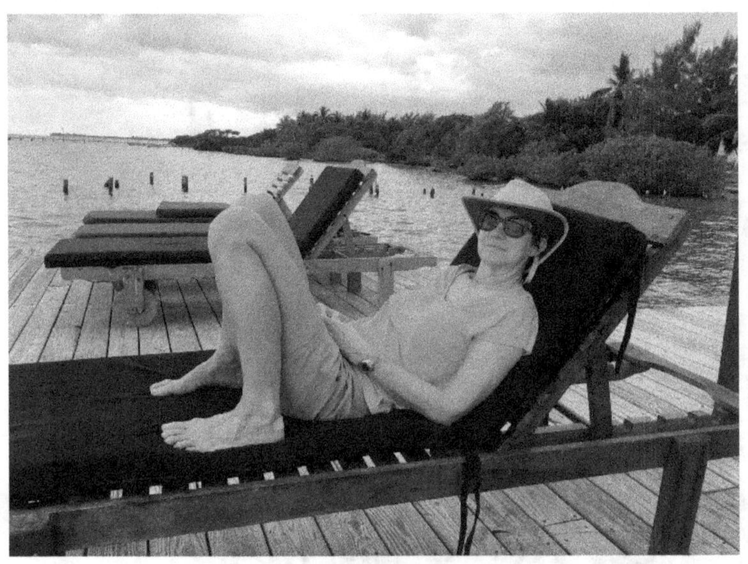

On the dock in Belize, 1/27/2019

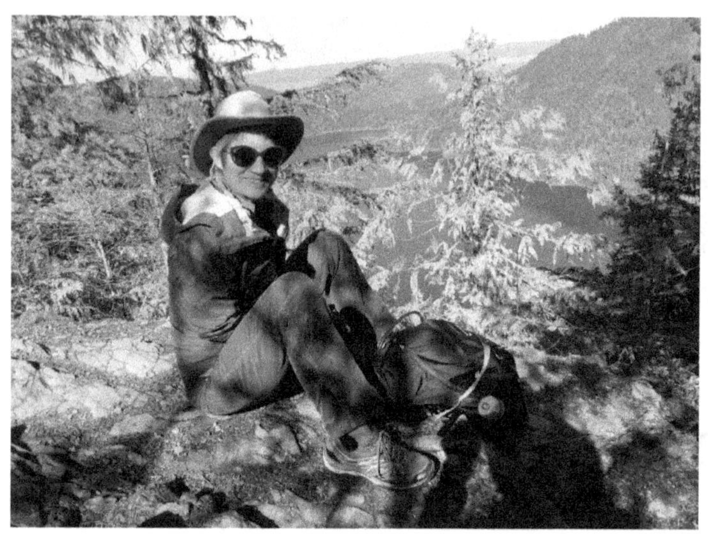

Olympic National Park, 10/6/2018

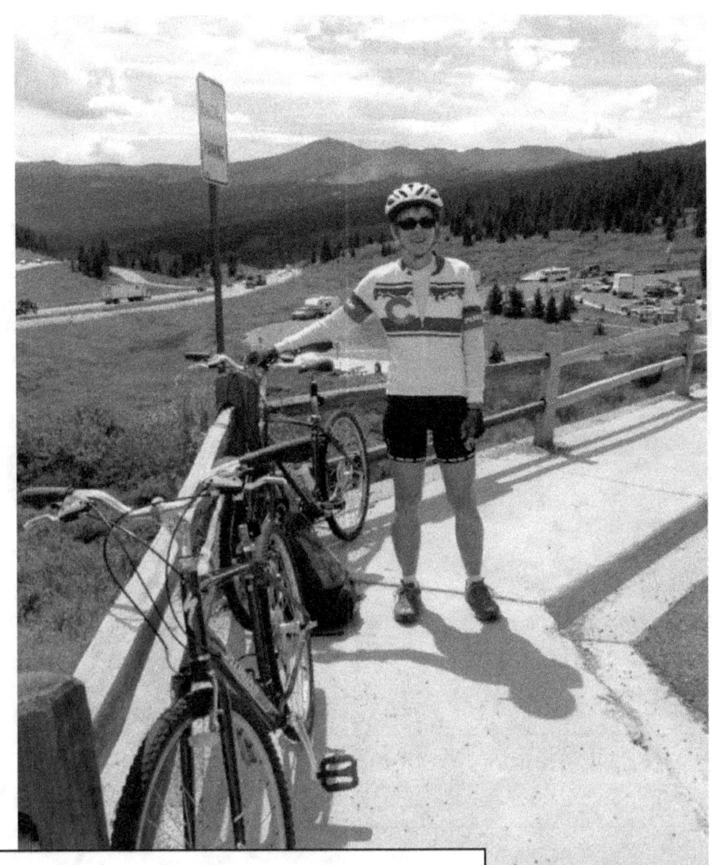

Dana at Vail Pass, after riding up 8/6/2013

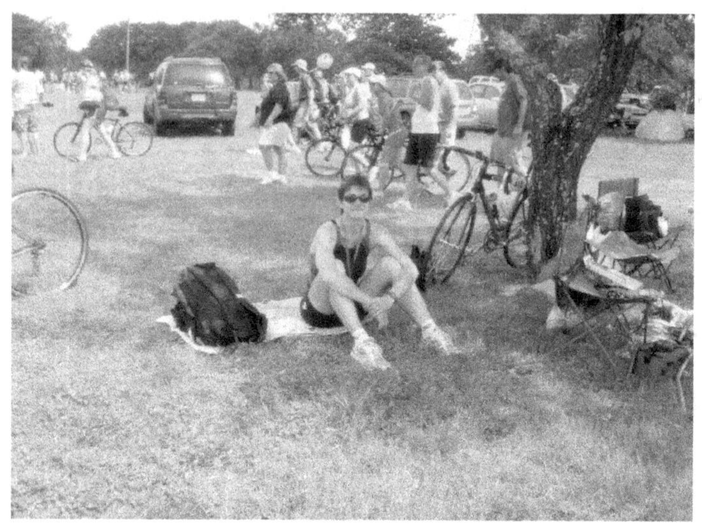

Dana after All Women's Triathalon, Austin, 6/10/2007

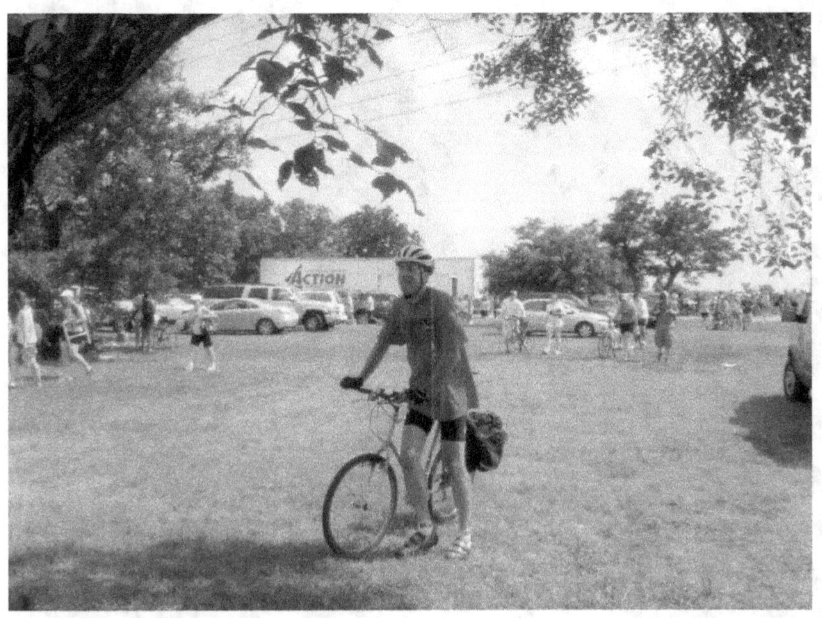

Britton after helping with the bikes at the All Women's Triathalon, Austin, 6/10/2007

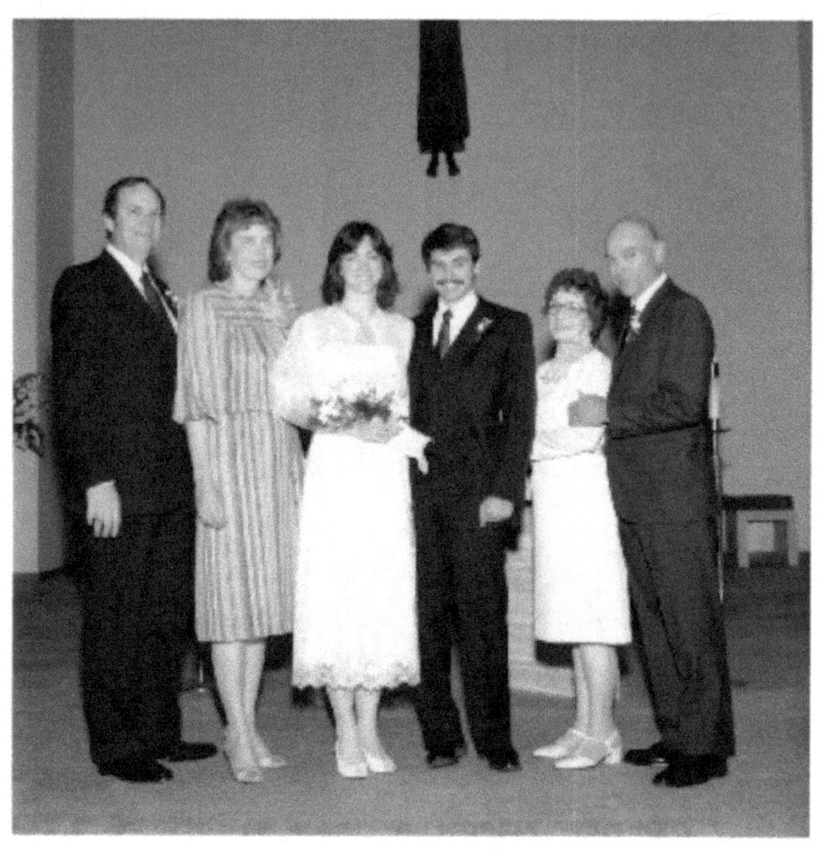

Wedding Picture with the Parents, March, 1983

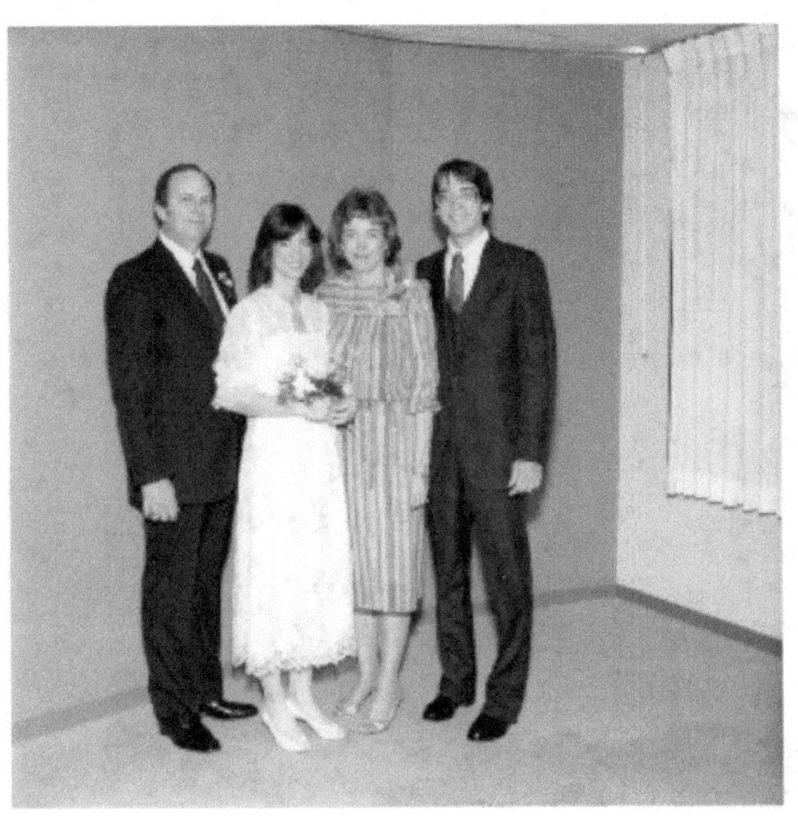

Guy, Dana, Dorothy and Britton Birmingham, March, 1983

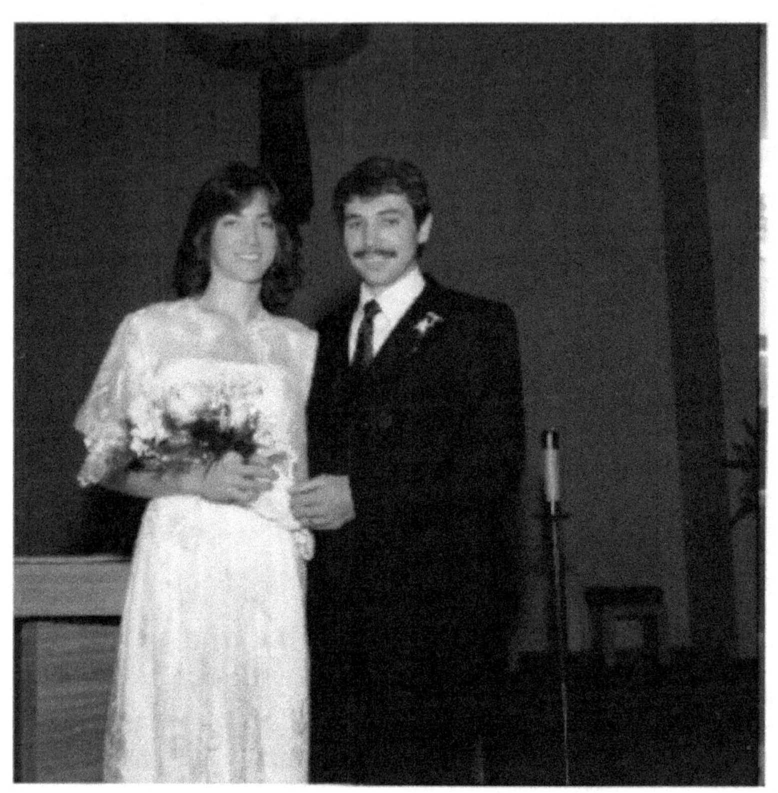